DATE OF RETURN
UNLESS RECALLED BY LIBRARY

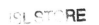

Health Promotion:
Professional Perspectives

USHEFMED

Health Promotion

Professional Perspectives

Edited by

Angela Scriven

and

Judy Orme

First published 1996 by
MACMILLAN PRESS LTD
Houndmills, Basingstoke, Hampshire RG21 6XS
and London
Companies and representatives
throughout the world

ISBN 0–333–64496–4 hardcover
ISBN 0–333–64497–2 paperback

A catalogue record for this book is available
from the British Library

10 9 8 7 6 5 4 3 2 1
05 04 03 02 01 00 99 98 97 96

Printed in Great Britain by
Antony Rowe Ltd, Chippenham, Wiltshire

Contents

Section three: Local authority

Section Four: Education and youth organisations

Section Five: Voluntary

Section Six: Workplace

List of figures and tables

Figures

Tables

The contributors

Lee Adams is Director of Health Promotion for Sheffield Health Authorities, and a member of the Healthy Sheffield Board. Her career spans 20 years, and includes being chair of the Society of Health Education/Promotion Specialists, a Director at the Health Education Authority and membership of the National Executive of the Family Planning Association. She is author of numerous publications.

Peter Allen is Head of Environmental Health at Oxford City Council and a Member of Green College, Oxford. He has written and lectured extensively on health promotion in local government.

Yvonne Anderson is a freelance education and training consultant. Yvonne became freelance in 1990 after a career in teaching, lecturing and residential care work. She works with a variety of voluntary organisations, including Victim Support Wiltshire, and she also serves on a voluntary organisation's management committee.

Penny Astrop is an experienced health service manager, currently working with Oxfordshire Family Health Service Authority (FHSA). Penny previously worked as a health visitor, health promoter and primary care team development facilitator. She specialises in the management of change, multiprofessional and interagency working.

Alan Beattie's career as a practitioner and researcher in health promotion spans 20 years in the NHS, school and voluntary settings, as well as universities. Alan was involved in the development of health promotion courses and research projects at London University from 1977 to 1989. He has been Honorary Senior Research Fellow in Applied Social Science at the Centre for Health Research at Lancaster University since 1989, becoming Head of Health Studies and Human Sciences at St Martin's College, Lancaster, in 1993, where he is now Professor in Health Promotion.

Marc Beishon is a freelance editor and writer. He has written regularly for *Healthlines*, the Health Education Authority's health promotion magazine, on a wide range of 'the health of the nation' topics. He has also carried out assignments on the information technology and publishing industries, as well as the education sector. Previously, he was managing editor of *New Scientist* magazine.

Jon Bloomfield, an economic and social historian by training with a PhD in post-war Czechoslovak history, has worked in local government in Coventry and Birmingham for the last decade. He is currently responsible for editing Birmingham's Community Care and Child Services plans and he coordinates the local authority's relations with all parts of the city's health services.

Sally Crowe is a Senior Health Promotion Specialist at South Buckinghamshire Health Promotion Service. After ten years' nursing experience and a spell in adult education, she moved into health promotion in 1991, specialising in workplace health issues. She currently works in sexual health, but maintains an interest in the development of workplace health promotion programmes.

Faith Delaney is a Senior Lecturer at Leeds Metropolitan University. She previously worked in local government and in the health service, as a nurse, researcher and health promotion specialist. She has experience of teaching and training with a wide range of occupational groups. She has published on intersectoral collaboration, health promotion in nursing and inequalities in child health. Research interests include public health strategy, evaluation and health promotion theory.

Linda Ewles is Health Promotion Manager for Avon Health Commission. She has worked as a health promotion specialist for over 20 years, in the NHS and in higher education. She is the author of many published articles, but most notably, with Ina Simnett, of *Promoting Health – A Practical Guide*, now in its third edition.

Stephen Farrow is Public Health Professor at Middlesex University and a Director of Public Health in Barnet. Previous posts include director of a university institute which specialised in the evaluation of health care. He has worked extensively on a range of projects and has acted as a consultant for the World Health Organisation, as well as many other national and international organisations.

Miriam Glover has worked in health promotion since 1989, specialising in the workplace setting. She has worked for Somerset Health Authority, the Health Education Authority and South West Regional Health Authority. Miriam is currently Health Promotion Alliances Manager in Somerset.

Zoë Heritage is a freelance consultant and trainer. After working in Africa for a number of voluntary organisations, she joined the Health Education Authority's (HEA's) Primary Health Care Unit as the

Community Development Officer. She is now a freelance consultant and she sits on the management committees of several voluntary organisations. In 1994 she edited the Royal College of GP's publication *Community Participation in Primary Care.*

Robin Ireland set up his own consultancy in 1993 specialising in lifestyle events, research and training. He has spent more than 10 years in the leisure and health promotion industries and has a keen personal interest in physical activity.

Miriam Jackson is currently a Senior Youth Work Development Adviser with the National Youth Agency. She previously worked for the Council for Education and Training in Youth and Community Work as an adviser and as a youth worker in three different local education authorities' youth services. Her published work includes two videos-led training packs, Building Portfolios 1 and 2, *A Personal Training Adviser's Handbook* and *Holistic Approaches to Health Education in Youth Work.*

Linda Jones is Lecturer in Health and Wellbeing and Chair of the Health Programme Area in the School of Health and Social Welfare at the Open University. Her research interests focus on the early growth of statutory welfare services and contemporary health policy. Her recent publications include *The Social Context of Health and Health Work* (1994) and (as co-editor) *Health and Wellbeing: A Reader* (1993).

Sue Latter is Principal Lecturer in Health Promotion at the Nightingale Institute, London. She has worked as a nurse in both hospital and community settings. Her research interests and publications have focused on nurses' perceptions and practice of health promotion in hospital settings.

Jennifer Lisle is a physician with a professional background in public health, psychological medicine and occupational health. As Director of Joint Research and Health Advisers since 1985 she has worked with both public and private sector organisations on a wide range of workplace health issues, including employee mental health and the design of occupational health services. She is a Senior Visiting Fellow at City University..

Kate Marsden is the Consumer Relations Officer at University Hospital Queens Medical Centre NHS Trust. Until recently she was the Information Officer at the Nottingham Self-Help Team. She was a contributing editor to *Self-Help: An Annotated Bibliography 1983-1993* and various articles on self-help and information.

Jonathan McWilliam is a Consultant in Public Health Medicine and Director of Health Strategy with Oxfordshire FHSA. His main interests include developing the role of GPs and purchasers and unifying the policies of DHAs and FHSAs, including health promotion policy.

Jan Myers is Training and Development Working/Assistant Team Leader at the Nottingham Self-Help Team. She is a qualified social worker and has worked in the voluntary sector for about 15 years. She has contributed to Team publications and various articles for sector magazines.

Judy Orme is a Senior Lecturer in Health Promotion at the University of the West of England in Bristol. Her background is in health-related research at the University of Bristol. Current research interests are health promotion in general practice, women's health and physical activity patterns in young people.

Ann Payne is currently a member of Tailor Made Training, Director of the HEA Health Promoting College project, and Coordinator for the Health Promotion Wales (HPW) Healthy Colleges' project. Her background includes social work, nursing, teaching in further education and research. Publications include *Training on the Right Track* (1991).

Diana Sanders is a Chartered Counselling Psychologist, working in the Oxfordshire Mental Health Care NHS Trust and Oxford University. She has a background in health promotion and research and has published on health promotion in the workplace, smoking cessation, health promotion in primary care and women's health.

Angela Scriven is Course Director for the MSc in Health Promotion and Subject Leader for Health Studies and Health Education in the undergraduate modular degrees at Bath College of Higher Education. Research interests and publications are centred on health education in schools and, more recently, women's health.

Keith Tones is Professor of Health Education at Leeds Metropolitan University. He has been involved in postgraduate health education teaching for over 20 years, and has acted as a consultant for the World Health Organisation and many other international and national organisations. He has published extensively.

Sarah Veale is a Senior Policy Officer at the Trades Union Congress. Her main responsibilities are for individual employment rights and workplace health promotion. She is a member of the Government's 'The Health of the Nation' Workplace Steering Group. She has spoken extensively on the role of trade unions in workplace health promotion.

Cheryl Wright has 11 years' health visiting experience and is now a Senior Nurse Manager in Gwent. During 1993 and 1994 she carried out extensive research into adolescent health, collaborating closely with major purchasers and providers of primary health care services in Bath.

Acknowledgements

Special thanks to Sue Nancholas and Caroline Rubery for their assistance in compiling the original proposal for the book and to Tina Jolly for her diligence and patience in finalising the manuscript.

Introduction

Angela Scriven and Judy Orme

Health Promotion is increasingly recognised as a central activity of many professional groups. The Government acknowledged this in the White Paper *The Health of the Nation* (Department of Health, 1992) and called for the establishment of collaborative partnerships between the various agencies and organisations that promote health.

The establishment of these collaborative activities requires careful consideration. The Department of Health (1993) list of prerequisites for inter-agency or alliance work clearly points to the need for constructive communication and a full understanding of the structure, philosophy, constraints to and possibilities for health promotion in a range of professional spheres of work.

There are a number of inherent difficulties associated with the promotion of health through collaborative partnerships. The notion that the advent and advancement of *healthy alliances* would be easily translatable at a local level, is based on a false premise.

The success of interagency health promotion initiatives is dependent on numerous factors. A key issue is undoubtedly the differing interpretations and ideological understanding of the term *health promotion* that the various agencies, and their respective representatives, espouse. Too frequently, the dominant strategy used is high profile events based on a narrow, rather than an holistic, view of health promotion practice. Approaches which encompass the full range of paradigms and are underpinned by a clear understanding of the principles of health promotion might require some professional groups to make uncomfortable shifts in ideology.

Another tension is that collaborative working is espoused as a cost-effective way of providing health promotion, in that the outcomes are hoped to be more than the sum of the parts. However, funding considerations do not disappear when responsibility is devolved locally. In fact, key organisations and agencies frequently undergo substantial organisational and funding changes. Uncertainties surrounding future organisational structures and available funding for health promotion often mitigate against the formation of collaborative interagency partnerships.

The central purpose of this text, therefore, is to offer an extensive insight into a variety of professional perspectives on health promotion,

1

in order to facilitate the process of effective collaborative work between professionals drawn from different backgrounds, with different cultures and ideologies. The tensions, conflicts and rewards of alliance working will be discussed in the contexts of a wide variety of settings. Because of its approach, the book will appeal to a wide range of readers including the following specialist groups and students training to become members of these groups:

• Specialist health promotion officers;
• Nurses and health visitors;
• Professions allied to medicine such as physiotherapists;
• Social workers;
• Teachers/trainers/LEA health education coordinators;
• Environmental health officers;
• Specialists in public health medicine.

The book has been written to meet a recognised need. Most other texts are practical guides *or* theoretical works that examine health promotion from economic, social, political and philosophical perspectives. This book, in contrast, offers detailed information about the opportunities and constraints to health promotion within a variety of professional contexts and examines how these are addressed, thus identifying diversity of practice. The text moves beyond rhetoric, therefore, by providing theoretical perspectives alongside accounts of practice.

The book consists of carefully selected contributions from a distinguished group of academics and health professionals in the UK. The list of more than 20 authors includes representatives from specialist health promotion, health services, local authorities, voluntary organisations and education.

The text is divided into six sections reflecting, for the most part, the professional settings within which health promoters operate. However, the settings are not seen as exclusive or definitive. It is recognised that some professionals work across settings. For the purposes of this book, for example, school nurses appear in the education and youth setting even though as a professional group, they are employed by the health service.

Moreover, education has not been incorporated into the local authority setting. The contributions within the education and youth setting are much wider than local authority, as they include the European health promoting schools initiative and 'The Health Promoting Colleges Project'.

Each section, therefore, has a specific focus and the coherence is provided by the complementary nature of the contributions.

Section one is the portion of the book which deals with a number of issues involving the integration of theory and practice that have relevance to the consideration of health promotion in different professional settings. How differing professional ideologies will influence the fundamental understanding of health and how it is best promoted is considered by Keith Tones in the opening chapter of the book. This chapter offers a broad analysis of the concept of health promotion and the importance of the synergistic relationship between education and healthy public policy. He suggests that essential questions need to be asked when considering working in particular settings.

An exploration of the possibilities and constraints to health promotion pervades the text. The efficacy of working across professional boundaries receives special attention by Faith Delaney in Chapter 2. The conceptual basis of intersectoral collaboration is discussed in depth and an overview is provided of the potential and pitfalls of alliance work in the current context of national policy, notably *The Health of the Nation*. These two chapters form the first section of the book and establish the theoretical issues that permeate the chapters that follow.

Section two of the book focuses on the health service and reflects the wide range of professional activities that are a feature of health promotion practice within this sector. The section begins with an overview of the implications for health promotion of the recent National Health Service (NHS) reforms. Lee Adams examines the complex process of purchasing and providing. The specific references made to Sheffield Health Authority provide a realistic assessment of the constraints and opportunities for health promotion in the wake of the NHS reforms.

Penny Astrop and Jonathon McWilliam add to this debate by providing a lively discussion of the changing role of the Family Health Service Authority (FHSA). The pivotal role of FHSAs in facilitating health promotion work in primary health care is highlighted and the autonomy that these authorities have to develop their own priority areas is assessed.

Judy Orme and Cheryl Wright follow this introduction to primary health care by considering the changes in delivery of health promotion in general practice over the last five years. This chapter sets out to illustrate how opportunities for innovative health promotion exist within a seemingly narrowly focused banding system. The role of community nurses is discussed, focusing on health visitors as key partners with general practitioners (GPs) in the development of appropriate health promotion in general practice.

Linda Ewles adds to this analysis by taking the reader through the fundamental and rapid changes within specialist health promotion in the NHS. These are considered under broad areas of organisational change and opportunities and constraints in the contract culture. An assessment is made of the relationship between health promotion specialists and public health medicine, and the current emphasis on efficiency and effectiveness is debated.

Sue Latter concludes this section by providing a detailed exploration of opportunities available for health promotion in hospital nursing practice. The nurses' specific role as health educators with patients is reviewed, followed by a critical analysis of the nurses' potential for collaborative health promotion partnerships. Constraints which may militate against achievement of this potential are highlighted.

Section three includes three chapters concentrating on the health promotion work of local authorities. Contributions centre on the development of health promotion within this sector at both local and national levels.

Peter Allen initiates this debate with an evaluation of the extent that environmental health services engage in health promoting activities, and an assessment of how the discretionary powers of environmental health officers can be used to this end. The implications for the newly forming unitary authorities are scrutinized in relation to the potential and constraints to health promotion within this professional sphere.

Following on from this, Linda Jones and Jon Bloomfield consider the potential for promoting health in the very pressured realm of social service provision. The barriers of a defensive culture are taken into account and links are made with all aspects of social service provision. The potential for collaborative work between social services and primary health care is explored in some detail.

Robin Ireland emphasises the connections between sport and health, by considering the roles of the Sports Council, the Health Education Authority (HEA) and local authorities. The potential for alliances between local authorities, primary health cre and the community are explored in some detail and the theoretical aspects of participation in sport and the role for health promotion are discussed.

Section four is concerned with the range of health promoters who operate within the education and youth-work professional domain. Angela Scriven raises major issues concerned with the delivery of health education in schools. The discussion on the impact of Government education policy focuses on the marginalisation of health education within the national curriculum framework, the decline of teacher advisers and the demise of health education in initial teacher training. Alan Beattie follows this with a fascinating analysis of the concept of the health promoting school, using the application of many recognised models or frameworks of health promotion.

The opportunities and strengths of the school nurse as a health promotion agent are examined by Stephen Farrow. The vulnerability of this particular group of health promoters is discussed in some detail. The potential for health promotion in further education is discussed by Ann Payne who draws on her involvement in the Health Promoting Colleges Project. Miriam Jackson concludes this section by identifying the tremendous potential within youth settings for health promotion. Examples of good practice across the country are highlighted.

Section five focuses on voluntary organisations. Yvonne Anderson and Zoë Heritage provide an overview of the opportunities for health promotion within this setting. The impact of recent legislation, organisational structures and funding pressures are highlighted as important considerations for health promoters. A case study of victim support is incorporated into this appraisal. The concept of self-help is explored by Jan Myers and Kate Marsden. The key issues of mutual support and active alliances with professionals are central to this discussion.

Section six considers health promotion within the workplace and is introduced by Diana Sanders and Sally Crowe who provide a thorough review of health promotion initiatives in the workplace. The importance of collaborative working is illustrated by using evidence from the literature and from case studies. Miriam Glover also uses a case-study approach to illustrate the real dilemmas and practicalities of setting up healthy alliances in the workplace setting. The important role of the trade unions in promoting health is examined by Marc Beishon and Sarah Veale. The underlying premise here is that the place for trade unions is as a part of any process involving decisions that will affect the health and well-being of employees. The final chapter of the book is written by Jennifer Lisle who focuses on the role of occupational health services, exploring opportunities for health promotion in the context of organisational structure. Analysis centres on the need for these services to adopt a proactive role in developing appropriate organisational strategies to support healthy organisations.

It is hoped that this volume will provide readers with a number of new insights into the diverse range of initiatives and activities that have come to be known as health promotion. Although many of the professional contexts in which health is promoted encompass constraints as well as possibilities for health promotion, the analysis of these provides a greater understanding of the scope for action and, of course, the possibility for collaborative endeavour.

References

Department of Health (1992). *The Health of the Nation*. London: HMSO.
Department of Health (1993). *Working Together for Better Health*. London: HMSO.

Issues concerned with theory and practice

1 The anatomy and ideology of health promotion: empowerment in context

Keith Tones

This chapter will provide an analysis of the concept of health promotion which is mainly based on the formulation which the World Health Organisation (WHO) has developed, largely since the launch of the movement to achieve *Health for All by the Year 2000* (*HFA2000*) at the 30th World Health Assembly in 1977. Both ideological and functional aspects of health promotion will be identified and, more particularly, its commitment to empowerment will be discussed. The importance of the potentially synergistic relationship between education and healthy public policy will also be emphasised. The implications of these various key features of health promotion for professional practice in a number of key settings and contexts will then be explored.

The meaning of health promotion

Health promotion is an essentially contested concept. It has been used in a variety of ways by different individuals and organisations, typically in the context of special pleading or in support of some cherished viewpoint or philosophy. Indeed, Green and Raeburn (1988) provide a rather useful description of the ways in which various individuals and groups have made their bids for ownership:

> Ideologues, professionals, interest groups, and representatives of numerous disciplines have attempted to appropriate the field for themselves. Health and education professionals, behavioral and social scientists, holistic health and self-care advocates, liberals, conservatives, voluntary associations, funding agencies, governments, community groups, and many others all want something from health promotion, all want to contribute something, and all bring their own orientation to bear on it. (p.30)

A comprehensive account of health promotion and its history is beyond the scope of this chapter and more complete analyses may be found elsewhere (for example, Anderson, 1984; Tones, 1985; Minkler, 1989). In this chapter, however, the definition adopted is substantially that of the WHO and we will, therefore, seek to tease out its essential features. We should, then, note the following important milestones marking progress from the 1977 initiation of *HFA2000*.

At one level, it could be argued that the roots of health promotion are to be found in the WHO's original and classic definition of health (World Health Organisation, 1946) with its holistic emphasis on well-being. It is, on the other hand, important to also note the change of emphasis embedded in *HFA2000*: health is no longer viewed as the ultimate purpose of health promotion but rather as a means to an end. The final goal is now conceived as a 'socially and economically productive life'. Clearly, this begs the question about the nature of social and economic productivity but is, nonetheless, a rather more manageable concept than perfect well-being!

Undoubtedly the most obvious precursor to health promotion is the Declaration of Alma Ata (World Health Organisation, 1978) which, *inter alia*, asserted that the existence of gross inequalities between advantaged and disadvantaged peoples was 'politically, socially and economically' unacceptable. The proposed solution to this problem was to be primary health care. This is not to be confused with primary *medical* care since demedicalization was to be an important thrust of primary health care (PHC) and, subsequently, health promotion. Moreover, given the perspective of the present book, we should also acknowledge how Alma Ata popularised the notion of intersectoral collaboration, which would later, in the UK, find a somewhat new expression in a recognition of the value of healthy alliances.

If Alma Ata and PHC were the prototypes, the emergence of health promotion as a kind of militant wing of *HFA2000* was formalised with the publication by the WHO's European Region of the concepts and principles in 1984. Kickbusch (1986) described this event as '... *a new forcefield for health* [which] *integrates social action, health advocacy and public policy*'. Arguably, the first full blossoming of the principles incorporated in the 1984 publication was to take place in Ottawa when 200 delegates from 38 nations made a commitment to health promotion in what has, since that time, been celebrated as the Ottawa Charter (World Health Organisation, 1986; *Health Promotion*, 1986). The specific features of the Charter may be consulted elsewhere and its principles will feature in the more extended review which is presented below. It is, though, worth noting that although reference was made to the importance of developing people's personal skills, health education was dislodged from the centre-stage position it enjoyed under the aegis of PHC and the new imperative was to be building healthy public policy. Perhaps the other most important ideological principle to emerge from Ottawa was its reiteration that the empowerment of individuals and communities should be a major focus of future work: community action must be strengthened and decision making facilitated by creating supportive environments. The theme of demedicalisation was also maintained and found expression in the argument for *reorientation of health services* in order to both expand their scope and make them more user-friendly.

Health promotion's progress was maintained both by attempts to activate the 38 targets for achieving *HFA2000* (World Health Organisation, 1985) and a number of subsequent conferences and major initiatives. For instance, a second international conference on health promotion was held in Adelaide (*Health Promotion*, 1988) which pursued ways of building healthy public policy and, most recently, a third international conference was held in Sundsvall (World Health Organisation, 1991). The Sundsvall Declaration focused on the need to provide supportive environments for health and highlighted four aspects: (i) the social dimension (the impact of cultural norms and social processes), (ii) the political dimension (requirement of governments to guarantee democratic participation in decision making and make a commitment to human rights and peace, (iii) the economic dimension (need to re-channel resources to achieve *Health for All*) and (iv) the need to recognise women's skills and knowledge.

In addition to the conferences and declarations, attempts to translate rhetoric into practice are specially relevant to the aims of this book. Perhaps the most significant of these was the Healthy Cities movement, which initially sought to establish test-beds for health promotion in 11 European cities. A more extended discussion of Healthy Cities may be consulted elsewhere (for instance Fryer, 1988 and Kickbusch, 1989). Suffice it to say that this WHO inspired development acted as a stimulus for the emergence of more than 300 local initiatives in various European cities. In addition to the focus on the city, the principles of health promotion were applied to a number of more specific institutions or organisations. Perhaps the most noteworthy of these has been the discovery of the health promoting hospital and the re-discovery of the health promoting school.

Key principles of health promotion

Two kinds of principle will be listed below. The first kind may be termed ideological and derives from the value position held by its advocates. In short, an ideological principle will state what the purpose of health promotion *ought* to be, as a kind of moral imperative. The second variety may be called functional in that each particular principle is best viewed as a means to the moral end. However, since these two aspects will often be embodied in one form of words, they will not be separately identified here. They may be summarised as follows:

- *Health*   Health should be viewed holistically and its positive aspect (that is, well-being) should be acknowledged. However, it should not be primarily considered as an end in its own right but rather as a means to an end; that is, the achievement of a socially and economically productive life.
- *Equity*   Inequalities between and within nations are intrinsically unacceptable; moreover, the achievement of preventive medical outcomes and health gain generally will be in proportion to governments' success in ensuring a more equitable distribution of resources.
- *Healthy public policy*   Since the major determinant of health and illness is the physical, cultural and socioeconomic environment in which people live and work, a narrow *individualistic* focus on personal responsibility is to blame the victim of these macro-level circumstances. Accordingly, *building healthy public policy* in order to create a supportive environment and make the healthy choice the easy choice is perhaps the most important single purpose of health promotion.
- *Reorientation of health services*   Health is too important to be left to the medical profession (and professions allied to medicine). There must be a reorientation of health services. Since medical services often do not meet population needs and are often depowering, they should be reformed. Demedicalisation is an important goal of health promotion: it is concerned not only to shift the balance of power from doctors and the medical establishment towards patients and clients, but it also seeks to acknowledge the substantial contributions which other services make to health (and illness). Services such as housing, transport, leisure and recreation, and economic development, may all influence health for good or ill. Healthy alliances based on efficient intersectoral collaboration should be established so that the health promoting potential of these services might be harnessed for the public good.
- *Empowerment*   The achievement of active participating communities is a prime goal of health promotion. Empowerment is worth pursuing in its own right, as a sign of individual and social health. It is also an essential means to ensure that individuals and communities will be able to make healthy choices and work proactively to enhance public health generally. Empowering strategies and tactics should operate in all situations and at all levels. The purpose of health education is, therefore, to raise critical consciousness,

provide supportive health skills and facilitate cooperation rather than compliance.

The contribution of education

Only the briefest of discussions about the relationship between health education and health promotion is possible here (for a more thorough review, see Tones and Tilford, 1994). In brief, health education is not synonymous with health promotion. It is, however, a major component within the wider scheme of things and makes a substantial contribution to the achievement of health promotion goals. Without health education the purposes of health promotion are unattainable. It is, arguably, most useful to think of there being a synergistic relationship between health education and one of the key constructs identified in the Ottawa Charter as *healthy public policy*. The relationship is probably multiplicative; that is, without the support of policy measures (which would result, for instance, in legislative or economic outcomes), education alone would achieve but limited success. On the other hand, without health education, it would be difficult if not impossible to overcome the various political obstacles with which vested interests confront attempts to implement health policies. The Ottawa Charter, on the other hand, set great store by lobbying strategies, the use of advocacy and mediation between conflicting interests in order to trigger political commitment to healthy public policy. As mentioned earlier, health education was marginalised. This confidence in the power of political lobbying is misplaced and it is, therefore, important that we be clear about the precise contribution which education might make to achieving Health for All. The key components of a health education strategy designed to make such a contribution are summarised as follows:

- Individually focused education designed to empower and facilitate decision making; its purpose is to provide support and achieve cooperation rather than to coerce, persuade and gain compliance.
- Individually focused education designed to promote judicious use of health and medical services. It includes assertive interaction with health practitioners.
- Community focused education designed to achieve critical consciousness raising (CCR), empowerment and, subsequently, political action leading to the implementation of healthy public policy at national, local and organisational levels.

An empowerment model of health promotion

The concept of empowerment is complex and, as with health promotion, it comprises an amalgam of ideological and technical attributes.

A full discussion is not, therefore, possible here and a more complete analysis may be found elsewhere (Tones, 1992, 1994; Tones and Tilford, 1994). *Figure 1.1* seeks to demonstrate the relationship between empowerment, health education and the attainment of health.

In short, two interrelated varieties of empowerment contribute ultimately to the achievement of health status. As we have seen, an active participating community is an essential goal of health promotion. Such a community will comprise the sum of empowered individuals within that community, and the purpose of an 'empowerment' approach to health education is to support both self-empowerment and community empowerment. Clearly, an empowered community will also generate norms and a social support system which will reinforce the process.

The net gain from empowerment will be the achievement of healthy public policy which achieves control over social and environmental circumstances. *Figure 1.1* thus demonstrates one of the central tenets of social learning theory which is embodied in the concept of reciprocal determinism (Bandura, 1982, 1986). In short, people's capacity for action (and ultimately their health) is determined by the nature of their environment; on the other hand, however, it is usually possible

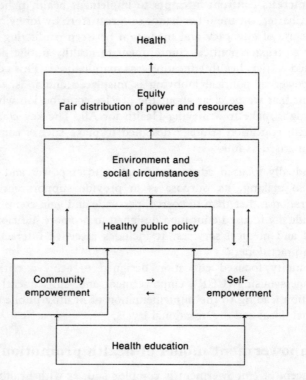

Figure 1.1   *Health education, empowerment and health promotion*

for people to exercise at least some degree of control over their circumstances. The relationship between the environment and the individual is thus one of reciprocity, except for those individuals who are continually overwhelmed by so many negative events and oppressive circumstances that their degree of choice is effectively zero.

I have defined empowerment elsewhere (Tones, 1994) as follows:

> Empowerment is a state in which an individual actually possesses a relatively high degree of power: that is having the resources which enable that individual to make genuinely free choices. Power cannot be absolute – and even if it could, it would be undesirable since it would militate against the right of other people to make choices. Indeed, one of the key features of empowerment is that system of checks and balances which safeguards the rights of others.
>
> Individual empowerment is associated with certain beneficial psychological characteristics of which the most significant are: beliefs about personal control – including realistic causal attributions – together with a relatively high level of self esteem based on a realistic self concept; valuing other people and their rights to self determination; possession of a repertoire of 'health and lifeskills'.
> (p.169)

Figure 1.2 illustrates the relationship between some of these factors and seeks to indicate how specific educational methods, such as group work, role play and modelling, might be deliberately used to influence the empowerment process.

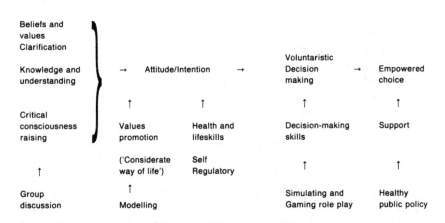

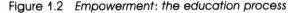

Figure 1.2 *Empowerment: the education process*

As we well know, the provision of knowledge is a necessary though insufficient prerequisite for achieving educational goals. It must be supplemented by the all-important process of critical consciousness raising which seeks not only to generate a state of heightened and critical awareness, but also to create indignation and concern over social issues and injustices. Those familiar with the philosophy of Freire (1972) will more fully appreciate the purpose of critical consciousness raising and its associated methodology. In one form or other it should be central to the overall health education enterprise.

However, apart from knowledge and raised awareness, people must actually believe they are capable of achieving their goals. As Bandura (*op. cit.*) demonstrated, they need both specific self-efficacy beliefs and, ideally, the conviction that they are in general in charge of their destiny (a state of mind associated with Rotter's (1966) well known construct, perceived locus of control).

Before individuals can freely choose and make empowered choices, they need a number of action competences (often described as health and lifeskills). These competences include a number of social interaction skills in addition to specific psychomotor skills which might be needed, for example, to adopt safe and effective exercise regimes. Some of the more frequently described lifeskills have to do with relaxation, time management and assertiveness. Self-regulatory skills, on the other hand, draw on the long-established tradition of behaviour modification which has increasingly been exploited to help people control difficult decisions and their sequelae, typically the loss of gratification and gain in discomfort from quitting unhealthy practices such as smoking or excessive alcohol consumption.

We should, of course, be aware that empowerment does not mean that 'anything goes'! As *Figure 1.2* shows, health promotion must involve an active process of values promotion in order to influence attitude and intention. The values in question will, of course, include those mentioned already as part of health promotion's ideological underpinning, concern for others, indignation at injustice and commitment to genuine democratic processes.

As will be readily apparent, the model in *Figure 1.2* concentrates on the educational rather than the policy aspect of health promotion: the important complementary feature of healthy public policy is merely signalled. We have, however, already emphasised that empowered choices are only possible when social and environmental factors support the individual choice. However, a discussion of policy formulation and implementation is beyond the scope of this chapter. The reader is, therefore, invited to note that a detailed set of principles derived from theory and practice could be formulated to considerably expand the minimalist representation which is featured in *Figure 1.2*.

Health promoting settings and contexts

I have thus far attempted to provide a particular framework which incorporates major features of health promotion with special reference to the importance of empowerment. The implications of this are doubtless obvious. If we subscribe to these health promotion principles, then we would expect to see them applied within all those settings and contexts in which attempts are made to promote people's health. Before providing a somewhat cursory review of what this might involve, it is worth providing a reminder that at least some of the many reviews of the function and management of health services in general have reached conclusions very similar to those adopted by the WHO. One of the best known examples is Maxwell's (1984) argument that a health care system should have six main dimensions: *accessibility, relevance, effectiveness, equity, acceptability* and *efficiency.* For further discussion of these similarities, Rathwell (1994) might usefully be consulted. *Inter alia,* he has pointed out that all six dimensions relate to the WHO's four dimensions of health gain: *equity, adding years to life, adding health to life,* and *adding life to years.*

Although often used interchangeably, the terms strategy, setting and context have different connotations (Tones, 1993). Strategy will be used here to refer to deliberate interventions which may or may not involve activities in different settings. Setting will, on the other hand, refer primarily to institutional locations – such as school or workplace. There is probably little difference between setting and context, but the latter might be more beneficially applied to situations such as community development where an educational process emerges in a given context. The notion of setting, on the other hand, does have a flavour of planned delivery.

At a strategic level, the peculiar characteristics and the benefits and disadvantages of particular settings should be itemised prior to calculating the contributions which they might make to an overall coordinated programme. As Whitehead and Tones (1990) have observed, this process may be assisted by asking five fundamental questions:

- *The question of access* What kind of target group may be accessed through a given setting? How many people will be reached and to what extent is their state of learning-readiness compatible with programme aims?
- *The question of philosophy and purpose* To what extent is the overall goal and philosophy of the setting compatible with the programme's philosophy and purpose?
- *The question of commitment* How committed is the organisation and its members to the programme goals?

- *The question of credibility* How credible is the institution and those within it who will be expected to act as health promoters? How will the public respond to them?
- *The question of competence* Irrespective of commitment and credibility, do the potential health educators and health promoters possess the knowledge and skills needed to communicate with and educate clients within the setting?

Settings and strategies: a selective review

In addition to gaining satisfactory responses to the five questions listed above, effective and ethical health promotion will also need to demonstrate the two ideological and functional principles discussed earlier in this chapter. Partly for ethical reasons but mainly in the interest of achieving effective outcomes, any given setting or strategy should be able to demonstrate that communication and education is enhanced by supportive healthy policy. Again, bearing in mind both ethical and efficiency issues, an empowerment approach should be adopted. Let us, therefore, at the risk of caricature, consider briefly some features of key strategies and contexts taking account of the above mentioned criteria.

- *The health promoting school* The nature of the health promoting school will receive full treatment in this book. We will merely note here how the long established concept of 'hidden curriculum' has been given new potency in the acknowledgement that teaching must be supported by healthy policy (for example, about food or personal relationships) if it is to bear fruit. Furthermore, we should acknowledge the fact that schools having effective personal and social education programmes are especially well placed to contribute to the attainment of the twin goals of CCR and empowerment.
- *The health promoting hospital* This most recent test-bed for health promotion is perhaps the most surprising and challenging, since hospitals have long been described as examples of total institutions which are virtually guaranteed to depower not only patients but any staff subservient to the medical profession! Recent initiatives do, however, seem to be in deadly earnest and insist that in order to join the club, the health promoting hospital must *inter alia: focus on health rather than disease; develop policy initiatives which ensure that the environment is health promoting and provide a model occupational health service; and actively empower both patients and staff.*
- *The workplace* Work-site health promotion is enjoying increasing popularity; indeed it has played a significant health promotion role in the US for many years. Bearing in mind that of the three key groups of actors (workers, trades union and managers), managers

are ultimately inspired purely by the profit motive when they allow health promoters to gain access to the workplace. Fortunately, all parties are likely to benefit from the cooperation, though the achievement of worker empowerment will doubtless not be accorded a very high profile! On the other hand, although the workplace may not be best placed to achieve consciousness-raising and empowerment goals, it does provide us with some of the best and most detailed examples and models of health policy development and implementation.

• *Primary care*   The primary care context is of special interest to the health promoter. Apart from the major advantage that the primary health care team can gain access to the practice population on a regular basis, it has at its disposal a credible and potentially skilled task force of health educators. However, although formally required (in the UK) to deliver health promotion, a quite substantial training task may be required to ensure that the educational encounter between doctor or nurse and patient are genuinely participatory. If recent work by Kendall (1993) is representative, involvement of clients is relatively uncommon! We might also note that health practitioners in primary care have a particular responsibility to try to provide social and environmental support for the healthy choices which their clients' wish to make. Although some scope may exist for enabling environmental improvement, it would be unreasonable to expect any individual health or education worker to tackle major social problems. The Ottawa Charter, however, reminds all health professionals of their potential advocacy function and the possibilities of lobbying for healthy public policy through professional associations.

• *Community development*   The central purpose of community development is to create an active participating community. It seeks to achieve a redistribution of power and resources in its concern with equity; it aims to raise critical consciousness, address the felt needs of a community and meet the empowerment goals at the heart of health promotion. At this point we will merely remind readers that many outreach programmes bear a superficial resemblance to community development in their informal work with disadvantaged communities. To the extent that their purpose is to impose a medical agenda in a top-down fashion on the community in question, their activities are better described as colonisation rather than empowerment! For a more complete review of the problematic nature of community development, see Tones and Tilford (*op. cit.*, chapter 8).

By way of conclusion, the obvious point to make is that maximum benefit will result from intersectoral work and a healthy alliance or coalition between all sectors and settings. It is also pertinent to reiterate the observation that through the synergistic operation of education and healthy public policy, health promotion seeks to empower choice and create an active and critical populace. In this way, hopefully, healthy choices will be easier to make than is the case at present. The goal is not to coerce but to foster personal growth and quality of life and, in so doing, reduce disease, premature death and disability.

References

Anderson, R. (1984). Health promotion: an overview. In *European Monographs in Health Education Research*, No. 6 (ed. L. Baric) Scottish Health Education Group, Edinburgh 4–126.

Backer, T. E., Rogers, E. M. & Sopory, P. (1992). *Designing Health Communications Campaigns: What Works?* Newbury Park: Sage.

Bandura, A. (1982). Self efficacy mechanism in human agency. *American Psychologist, 37*(2), 122–147.

Bandura, A. (1986). *Social Foundations of Thought and Action: A Social Cognitive Theory*. New Jersey: Prentice-Hall.

Durrant, K. (1992). Pedagogy of the Oppressed. In W. G. Bennis (ed.), *The Planning of Change*. New York: Holt.

Freire, P. (1972). *Pedagogy of the Oppressed*, Penguin, Harmondsworth.

Fryer, P. (1988). A healthy city strategy three years on – the case of Oxford city council. *Health Promotion, 3*(2), 213–218.

Green, L. W. & Raeburn, J. M. (1988). Health promotion. What is it? What will it become? *Health Promotion, 3*(2), 151–159.

Health Promotion (1986), *1*(4), the whole issue.

Health Promotion (1988). The Adelaide recommendations: healthy public policy. *Health Promotion, 3*(2), 183–186.

Kendall, S. (1993) Client participation in health promotion encounters with health visitors. In J. Wilson-Barnett & J. Macleod Clark, *Research in Health Promotion*. London: Macmillan.

Kickbusch, I. (1986). Issues in health promotion. *Health Promotion, 1*(4), 437–442.

Kickbusch, I. (1989) Healthy cities: a working project and a growing movement. *Health Promotion, 4*(2), 77–82.

Maxwell, R. (1984). Quality assessment in health. *British Medical Journal, 288*, 1470–1472.

Minkler, M. (1989). Health education, health promotion and the open society: an historical perspective. *Health Education Quarterly, 16*, 17–30.

Rathwell, T. (1994). Health care systems in the United Kingdom and Canada: can they deliver? In K. Lee (ed.), *Health Care Systems in Canada and the United Kingdom?* Keele: University Press.

Rotter, J. B. (1966). Generalised expectancies for internal versus external control of reinforcement. *Psychological Monographs, 80*(1), 1–28.

Tones, B. K. (1985). Health promotion: a new panacea? *Journal Institute of Health Education, 23*, 16–21.

Tones, B. K. (1992) Health promotion, empowerment and the concept of control. In *Health Education: Politics and Practice*. Victoria, Australia: Deakin University Press.

Tones, B. K. (1993). Changing theory and practice: trends in methods, strategies and settings in health education. *Health Education Journal, 52*(3), 126–139.

Tones, B. K. (1994). Health promotion, empowerment and action competence. In B. Jensen & K. Schnack (eds), *Action and Action Competence*. Copenhagen: Royal Danish School of Educational Studies.

Tones, B. K. & Tilford, S. (1994). *Health Education: Effectiveness, Efficiency, Equity*. London: Chapman & Hall.

Whitehead, M. & Tones, B. K. (1990). *Avoiding the Pitfalls*. London: Health Education Authority.

World Health Organisation (1946). *Constitution*. Geneva: WHO.

World Health Organisation (1978). *Report on the International Conference on Primary Health Care, Alma Ata, 6–12 September*. Geneva: WHO.

World Health Organisation (1984). *Health Promotion: a Discussion Document on the Concept and Principles*. Copenhagen: WHO.

World Health Organisation (1985). *Targets for Health for All*. Copenhagen: WHO.

World Health Organisation (1986). *Ottawa Charter for Health Promotion: An International Conference on Health Promotion, November 17–21*. Copenhagen: WHO.

World Health Organisation (1991). *Sundsvall Statement on Supportive Environments for Health, 9–15 June*. Geneva: WHO.

2 Theoretical issues in intersectoral collaboration

Faith Delaney

Health promoters have long recognised the importance of working together. The logic is indisputable: if health is more than the absence or treatment of disease, then its promotion and maintenance lie beyond the remit of any one professional group or sector. Intersectoral Collaboration has thus become a familiar term in health promotion. It is for the World Health Organisation (WHO) a key principle and central to achieving the goal of *Health for All by the year 2000* (World Health Organisation, 1984, 1985). 'Local Healthy Cities' and 'Health for All' (HFA) projects have proliferated, following the WHO's lead (Ashton, 1992; Tsouros, 1991). These are by definition intersectoral, resting on and generating collaboration at practice and policy levels. An ultimate goal is to develop 'healthy public policy' (World Health Organisation, 1986; Evers *et al.*, 1990).

The Health of the Nation strategy for England reinforces the importance of professionals working together, seeing 'Healthy Alliances' as a key vehicle for achieving its goals (Department of Health, 1992, 1993a). Alliances foster the involvement, and sense of ownership and commitment, of all those with an interest in health. The Secretary of State for Health has justified collaborative working by suggesting that through healthy alliances we can all achieve more than we would by working separately (Department of Health, 1993a).

Such justifications are familiar, both from practitioners and in literature on intersectoral collaboration. There is as yet no distinct body of literature or identifiable theory of collaboration. No area of professional practice can claim a monopoly on collaboration. Practitioners have their own well-developed ideas about what facilitates and hinders joint working. Yet, as Hudson has argued, despite widespread acknowledgement of the importance of collaboration to effective practice and policy:

> ...we know remarkably little about how [it] works, why it initially developed, how it may be measured or even how it may be defined.
> (Hudson, 1987, p.175)

In health promotion there is a growing consensus around features of successful collaboration. Experiences and impressions of professionals are supported by research studies. These have contributed to theorising about the organisational and interpersonal factors which impinge on collaboration. Useful concepts and metaphors can be identified in a wide range of disciplines such as psychology, organisational studies and social policy. This chapter will briefly comment on these and on recent studies into alliances, in considering the theory of collaboration. Of course, caution is important when producing and interpreting such summaries. Collaborative behaviour and policy development are complex and contingent human processes, and a single theory will probably remain elusive.

What would we expect a theory of collaboration to offer? It should at least offer insight into why collaboration occurs, how it is manifest, what inhibits or facilitates collaboration and, ultimately, what effect it has had. Practitioners use theory selectively, recognising that it may be partial, flawed or even inconsistent. Ultimately, theory should be of use in helping to understand a particular phenomenon and, as such, it should relate to experience.

Level of collaboration

There is a diversity of collaboration in practice. It can mean day-to-day liaison between health and social care professionals about clients, leading to 'seamless' care. In health promotion, it might involve ongoing liaison on issues of shared concern. Collaboration can also refer to new initiatives, where resources from a range of agencies are required or where funding is sought for a new multi-disciplinary project. As several commentators have noted, it is more rarely that coordination of policy across and within key agencies is sought (Springett, 1994).

How professionals with a health promotion remit work together depends to a large extent on the nature and purpose of an alliance. Alliances can be loose or formal, single-issue or broad-based, and they may have a fixed timescale or an ongoing remit for health issues.

In their research into healthy alliances within one English region, Nocon *et al.* (1993) noted so many different levels and degrees of collaboration that it was impossible to map them all. They presented a useful classification of types of alliance in one study which considered (geographical) *scope* from country through to neighbourhood. The *focus* of the work was classified as client group, such as children, or health issues, like nutrition. More comprehensively, the focus might be 'Health for All' (Office of Public Management, 1993).

The different *settings* or professional contexts, as outlined in this text, might be placed on either dimension. A network of school-based health promoters might exist across a district or county (see, for example, Chapter 12). Conversely, smoking cessation might be tackled by workplace health promoters (see Section 6). A local HFA or 'Healthy Cities' initiative will consult widely and develop a coordinated strategy (UK Health for All Network, 1993). However, the visible implementation of such a plan might be in the form of distinct projects on specific issues, for example mental health, or with client groups such as gay men. So there may be a myriad of smaller and more focused alliances within a 'parent' alliance at county, city or district level. Alongside health promotion projects, organisational change is encouraged to ensure that partner organisations prioritise health. The policies and procedures of such agencies should thus reflect health promotion principles.

Such a goal is more ambitious, difficult yet potentially rewarding. One study noted that the larger the geographical scale, the more partners are involved making the alliance more complex (Office of Public Management, 1993). A number of areas have started this process, notably with consultation and needs assessment and development of city-wide strategies (Adams, 1991, UK Health for All Network, 1993). Clearly, policy and organisational theories are relevant to this level of collaboration (see Pederson *et al.*, 1988; Walker, 1992; Health Education Unit LMU, 1993; Delaney, 1994a; Springett, 1994; and Farrant, 1994 for reviews which draw out implications for Health Promotion/Health For All).

Influences on collaboration

The majority of initiatives listed in *The Health of the Nation* documents have been at project level. While the level of operation of an alliance is important, the influences on collaboration operate at all levels. One way to classify the influences on collaboration is chronologically, from early days to maturity of an alliance (Gray, 1985; Butterfoss *et al.*, 1993).

Why professionals seek collaboration is of interest. Minimisation of client frustration and dwindling resources are the 'twin motives' often given as reasons for collaboration (Whetten, 1982). Resource availability depends on the general economic and political context but the impact of such factors is contested and difficult to establish objectively. Some studies and experiences suggest that cuts in funding can hinder collaboration (for example the removal of GEST funding discussed in Chapter 11). Yet other studies suggest that redirection of current resources could enable collaboration (Health Education Unit

LMU, 1993). Supporting this view, Hudson (1987) argues that in austere times collaboration increases. However, quality of collaboration can vary between local areas, despite the fact that they operate in the same national economic context (Delaney and Moran, 1991).

Specific central direction, legislation and formal requirements might initiate collaboration. In the British welfare context these have been rare. Furthermore, where the trend has been towards government directives, notably in joint care planning (Hardy *et al.*, 1990), this has not been particularly effective. The impact of recent government policy on collaboration in health promotion is discussed later.

So, incentives for professionals to work together might be negative, to fill a gap, or stem from a positive recognition of mutual need. In reality, no single factor would operate alone. However, in the formative stages one factor has repeatedly been identified as essential, and that is the sharing of a clear purpose. This is referred to by Gray (1985) as 'direction setting'. More recently, in the British context 'shared vision' is seen as central to collaboration and healthy alliances (Office of Public Management, 1993; Department of Health, 1993a; Health Education Unit LMU, 1993; LRC, 1993). Inability to come to consensus about goals and direction is one of the major frustrations in alliance building, particularly where different professional groups hold conflicting views of health and health promotion. This, in part, explains the importance of pre-existing networks with existing bonds and a shared history of successful collaboration (Gray, 1985; Zapka, 1992).

The source of the initial idea and the rationale provided are further considerations; are alliances developed as a response to national targets or in response to local health needs? What role has the community played in the decisions? Involvement is a well-established principle of ethical and effective health promotion. Furthermore, communication of innovations and change-management literature suggests that the urgency, relevance and tangibility of the problem affect the uptake of new approaches (Beardshaw *et al.*, 1990). This would need to be shared by the various groups involved.

In the maintenance stages of alliances, a range of significant factors have been identified. Resource commitment is important here too: resources might be informational, administrative or an input of time and skills. Injection of resources is seen as a key indicator of commitment, but this need not necessarily be on an equal basis. The degree of top-level support and the commitment of partner organisations are important factors. Basically, people work together if their needs are satisfied. Key factors which contribute to such satisfaction have been identified by Hudson (1987). 'Domain consensus' refers to agreement about areas of responsibility and boundaries of each organisation. Awareness of dependence on each other and similarity of function is necessary, otherwise the need to collaborate would not be perceived. Furthermore positive mutual awareness of those involved in an alliance is essential.

A second way to classify influences on collaboration is to distinguish between *structural* and *interpretive* factors (Halpert, 1982). Structural factors include the economic backdrop, as discussed, but also the way collaboration is organised. Most alliances develop an organisational structure with communication and reporting channels. While in Healthy Cities, a range of informal mechanisms have developed, there is a general view that a degree of formalisation is necessary, including statements of mission/philosophy, and formal procedures. Committee formation and clarification of roles is considered important as it justifies time and resource allocation. (UK Health for All Network, 1993; Curtice and McQueen, 1990).

Membership is an important consideration. Which professional and voluntary groups are represented can be very significant, to those included or excluded. Of particular note is where and how the community are represented in joint ventures. This may be determined by the impetus for the alliance, which to a large extent remains with the statutory sector. Professional dominance and protectionism can also cause problems: different groups may hold competing views about health and about participation. Smith (1988) outlines the importance of involving users at all stages, including decisions as to who should be involved, in her study of collaboration for mental health services. Consultation exercises for city-wide health strategies have explored community perceptions of health and need (UK Health for All Network, 1993). Voluntary and self-help groups also make a major contribution to health promotion (for further details see Chapters 16 and 17). Community involvement is important in respect of two other HFA principles : equity and participation.

A fundamental structural issue is the degree to which socioeconomic influences on health can be tackled locally, when decisions are increasingly made at international level. This is crucial for Healthy Cities (Kickbusch et al., 1990), although there may be limits to what health promoters can achieve together locally. Yet, health promotion emphasises empowerment and collective action. Alliances attempt in a variety of ways to address this dilemma. City-wide health initiatives often give central place to redressing inequalities. Other more modest alliances seek to improve the well-being of disadvantaged groups; for example, food cooperatives, black people's HIV/AIDS groups, accident prevention loan schemes, and so forth (Department of Health, 1993a).

In reality, the distinction between interpretive and structural factors is difficult to maintain. Many so called structural factors are in fact open to different interpretations. Costs and benefits, whether time spent is worthwhile, shared goals and values, the degree of control by any professional group, different views of health and so on are not objective facts but are dependent on the subjective views of health promoters. The interpersonal element in collaboration is well recognised. Regardless of the task, whether developing a strategy for purchasing for health gain or working on a multi-agency community drug project, similar issues arise. People need to feel positively valued, recognised and fully involved. Trust is at the heart of the microdynamics of collaboration (Webb, 1991).

This applies within professional settings as well as in joint alliances. Professional autonomy can have a positive or negative effect. 'Street level bureaucrat' describes workers with discretion who, for many reasons, might subtly resist new policies (Lipsky, 1976). This can apply wherever policy is developed in a 'top-down' way, again suggesting that health promotion policy will be more successful where full participation is valued.

Interorganisational and interpersonal networks

The term network is used very freely and in relation to several kinds of entity in health promotion. It is a key concept in the developing theory of collaboration. *Interorganisational network* usefully describes policy coordination locally and nationally (Means *et al.*, 1991) and could be extended to joint health promotion projects (Delaney, 1994a). A coordinating body or forum is often established and short-term ventures may be planned, but longer-term planning can also be undertaken (Harrison and Tether, 1987). Health for All networks are described as more fluid organisations (UK Health for All Network, 1993).

Social networks are groups of people upon whom we rely for socio-emotional or practical help (Hibbard, 1985). Furthermore, the social support that such networks provide is thought to confer health benefits (Dean, 1986), possibly by protecting us from or reducing stressful life events (Cohen and Syme, 1985). Work-related networks have beneficial effects on those involved. A study into health education certificate courses noted the importance of 'professional support networks' in fulfilling both social and professional development needs (Heathcote, 1991). The value of this process aspect of alliances has been identified in many recent studies (Office of Public Management, 1993; London Research Centre, 1993; Health Education Unit LMU, 1993; Delaney, 1994b). We noted earlier the centrality of trust to collaboration, and Springett (1994) suggests that such networks reflect innate needs to connect and affiliate.

Networking is clearly central to health promotion work across professional settings, to share information, improve coordination, to gain support and feel valued. Ability to network is one skill attributed to reticulists. These are staff who work at the boundaries between agencies and employ political astuteness and strategic thinking (Friend *et al.*, 1974; Sanderson, 1991; Health Education Unit LMU, 1993). However, other skills and characteristics are identified in recent studies of alliances: negotiation, credibility and patience, for example. The list is potentially overwhelming. However, most are skills that can be developed and, furthermore, they are skills increasingly required by the reflective practitioner in any setting.

The complementary notions of reticulist and network can provide a useful analogy for 'healthy alliances'. Springett (1994) sees networks at the interpersonal level as based on common values and information and bound by shared beliefs. The interorganisational network can be seen as a middle or 'meso'-level concept, linking the interpersonal and macro-structural levels (Delaney, 1994a). Springett correctly notes the need for further research into the interrelationship between networks at different levels.

Role of *The Health of the Nation* in fostering alliances

Power and control are not necessarily equitably distributed within society or within alliances. Commentators have noted the tendency in discussing intersectoral collaboration (ISC) to minimise conflict and maximise consensus (Research Unit in Health and Behavioural Change, 1989). This may smooth out fundamental and ideological differences between professionals and other stakeholders about appropriate interventions, thus protecting the status quo (Farrant and Taft, 1990). At this macro level of analysis, fundamental concerns reappear about equity, power and control over health chances.

These concerns underlie the questions to ask of *The Health of the Nation*. To what extent does it permit conditions for successful collaboration to develop, and what is the outcome of such collaboration? On what grounds are alliances deemed healthy?

By providing a high profile, an organisational framework and a national statement of health values, we could argue that this has contributed to a climate conducive to collaboration. By successfully achieving 'soundbite' status for the term *healthy alliance*, the principle of collaboration is legitimated throughout the NHS and beyond. The description of healthy alliance offered by the Department of Health (1993a, p.22), is borrowed from the following:

a partnership of individuals and organisations ... to enable people to influence the factors that affect their health and well-being, physically, mentally, socially and environmentally.

(Adams in OPM, 1993, p.4).

Many critics of *The Health of the Nation* White Paper have argued that a narrow, disease-oriented view of health is apparent. Furthermore, we can question the extent to which people are being enabled to influence multiple dimensions of health. How far does *The Health of the Nation* enable communities to influence their environment, be it socioeconomic or physical? The lack of incentive to professionals outside the health service and the weak position of health against more powerful sectors have been seen as major barriers to collaboration (Nocon *et al.*, 1993; Ewles, 1993; Delaney, 1994b). It has been asserted that to achieve health for *all*, we must 'threaten existing ... bureaucratic structures and professional empires, and ultimately the structures of society' (Farrant and Taft, 1990, p.137).

From such a perspective, incentives to collaborate, such as healthy alliance awards, seem at best inadequate. Nevertheless, despite initial scepticism, a substantial degree of activity has been undertaken – formally within the national implementation framework (Department of Health, 1993b) and locally with a good deal of local application and innovation. Nationally, there has been some progress towards policy appraisal and intra-governmental alliances for health, and there has been much local action within the professional contexts represented in this book. Clearly, criticism must be modified in the light of implementation experience. The chapters that follow note both the successes and the frustrations. Constant organisational change, as discussed in Section 2, and demands for cost containment suggest that the wider policy context still militates against working together for health gain.

Outcomes of collaboration

The debate will continue, in theory and practice. The theory of collaboration remains tentative and further research is required. Concepts will be refined, synthesising academic insight and practical experience. Meanwhile, health promoters will continue to collaborate and maintain their commitment to improving and redistributing health. While the increasing attention to process issues in alliances is welcome, ultimately, outcomes are the key concern. Alliances must be wary of the tendency for bureaucracies to become ends in themselves. The judgements of alliance members on their success are important but provide only one dimension, and the effectiveness of alliances should be reflected in their achievements. These issues are currently receiving attention (Speller and Funnell, 1993; Royston, 1993). Measuring health outcomes is a contentious issue but it is essential to evaluate collaborative health promotion work on criteria other than activity or disease targets. Then we might claim to have achieved healthy collaboration and healthy alliances.

References

Adams, L. (1991). *Healthy Sheffield 2000 Public Health Strategy.* Paper for WHO Euronet, Toulouse, France. September 1991.

Ashton, J. (ed.) (1992). *Healthy Cities.* Milton Keynes: Open University Press.

Beardshaw, V., Hunter, D. & Taylor, R. (1990). Power to prevent. *Health Service Journal* (25 January), 118–119.

Butterfoss, F. D., Goodman R. M. & Wandersman, A. (1993). Community coalitions for prevention and health promotion. *Health Education Research: Theory and Practice, 8*(3), 315–330.

Cohen, S. & Syme, S. L. (1985). (eds) *Social Support and Health.* Orlando: Academic Press.

Curtice, L. & McQueen, D. (1990). *The WHO Healthy Cities Project – An Analysis of Progress.* Working Paper No 40. Edinburgh: Research Unit in Health and Behavioural Change.

Dean, K. (1986). Social support and health: pathways of influence. *Health Promotion, 1*(2), 133–50.

Delaney, F. & Moran, G. (1991). Collaboration for health promotion: in theory and practice. *Health Education Journal, 50*(2), 97–99.

Delaney, F. (1994a). Muddling through the middle ground: theoretical concerns in intersectoral collaboration. *Health Promotion International, 9*(4), 217–223.

Delaney, F. (1994b). Making connnections: research into intersectoral collaboration. *Health Education Journal, 58* (forthcoming).

Department of Health (1991). *The Health of the Nation: A Consultative Document for Health in England.* London: HMSO.

Department of Health (1992). *The Health of the Nation: A Strategy for Health in England.* 1986. London: HMSO.

Department of Health (1993a). *Working Together for Better Health.* London: HMSO.

Department of Health (1993b). *The Health of the Nation One Year On.* London: HMSO.

Ewles, L. (1993). Hope against hype. *Health Service Journal* (July), 30–31.

Evers, A., Farrant, W. & Trojan, A. (eds) (1990). *Healthy Public Policy at Local Level.* Colarado: West View Press.

Farrant, W. (1994). Building healthy public policy: the healthy communities movement as an entry point. A review of recent literature. *Critical Public Health, 5*(1), 49–63.

Farrant, W. & Taft, A. (1990). Building healthy public policy in an unhealthy climate: a case study from Paddington and North Kensington. In A. Evers *et al., op. cit.*

Friend, J. K., Power, J. & Yewlett, C. (1974). *Public Planning: The Intercorporate Dimension.* London: Tavistock.

Gray, B. (1985). Conditions facilitating interorganisational collaboration. *Human Relations, 38,* 911–936.

Halpert, B. P. (1982). Antecedents. In D. L. Rogers & D. A. Whetten (eds), *Interorganisational Coordination: Theory, Research and Implementation*, 1st ed. Iowa: Iowa State University Press.

Hancock, T. (1990). Developing healthy public policy at local level. In A. Evers *et al.*, *op. cit.*

Hardy, B., Wistow, G. & Rhodes, R. A. W. (1990). Policy networks and the implications of community care policy for people with mental handicap. *Journal of Social Policy*, *19*(2), 141–168.

Harrison, L. & Tether, P. (1987). The coordination of UK policy on alcohol and tobacco: the significance of organisational networks. *Policy and Politics*, *15*(2), 77–90.

Health Education Unit, Leeds Metropolitan University (HEULMU) (1993). *Making Connections: Intersectoral Collaboration for Health*. Final report. Leeds: LMU.

Heathcote, G. (1991). *Networks: Their Role in the Professional Development and Support of Health Educators*. London: Health Education Authority.

Hibbard, J. H. (1985). Social ties and health status. *Health Education Quarterly*, *12*, 23–34.

Hudson, B. (1987). Collaboration in social welfare: a framework for aalysis. *Policy and Politics*, *15*, 175–182.

Hudson, B. (1989). Collaboration: the elusive chimera. *Health Services Journal* (January), *19*, 82–83.

Kickbusch, I., Draper, R. & O'Neill, M. (1990). Healthy public policy: a strategy to implement the Health for All philosophy at various governmental levels. In A. Evers *et al.*, *op. cit.*

London Research Centre (1993). *Healthy Alliances: A Study of Inter-agency Collaboration in Health Promotion*. South West Thames Regional Health Authority.

Lipsky, M. (1976). Towards a theory of street-level bureaucracy. In M. Lipsky *et al.*, *Theoretical Perspectives on Urban Politics*. Prentice-Hall, Englewood Cliffs: NJ.

Lukes, S. (1974). *Power: A Radical View*. London: Macmillan.

Means, R., Harrison, L., Jeffe, S. S. & Smith, R. (1991). Co-ordination, collaboration and health promotion: lessons and issues from an alcohol education programme. *Health Promotion International*, *6*(1), 31–40.

Milio, N. (1986). Multisectoral policy and health promotion: where to begin. *Health Promotion*, *1*(2), 129–132.

Mulford, C. L. & Rogers, D. L. (1982). Definitions and models. In D. L. Rogers & D. A. Whetten *op. cit.*

Nocon, A., Small, N., Ferguson, B. & Watt, A. (1993). Made in heaven? *Health Service Journal* (2 Dec), 24–26.

Office of Public Management (1993). *Healthy Alliances: Report to Standing Conference on Health Gain, 1992*. London: OPM.

Pederson, A. P., Edwards, R. K., Marshall, V. W., Allison, K. R. & Kelner, M. (1988). *Coordinating Healthy Public Policy. An Analytic Literature Review and Bibliography*. Canada: Health Service and Promotion Branch.

Rathwell, T. (1992). Pursuing health for all in Britain – an assessment. *Social Science and Medicine*, *34*(2), 169–182.

Rogers, D. L. & Whetten, D. A. (eds) (1992). *Interorganisational Coordination: Theory, Research and Implementation*. 1st ed. Iowa: Iowa State University Press.

Royston, G. (1993). A monitoring and evaluation framework for the implementation of 'the Health of the Nation'. In M. Malek, P. Vacani, J. Rasquina & P. Davey (eds), *Managerial Issues in the Reformed NHS*. London: John Wiley.

Research Unit in Health and Behavioural Change (RUHBC) (1989). *Changing the Public Health*. London: John Wiley.

Sanderson, I. (1990). *Effective intersectoral collaboration: the theoretical issues*. Working Paper 1, Intersectoral Collaboration and Health For All Project, Leeds Polytechnic.

Smith, H. (1988). *Collaboration for Change: Partnerships Between Service Users, Planners and Managers of Mental Health Services*. London: King's Fund Centre.

Speller, V. & Funnell, R. (1993). *Towards Evaluating Healthy Alliances*. HEA Multisectoral Collaboration for Health Evaluation Project, phase 1. HEA/ Wessex Institute of Public Health Medicine.

Springett, J. (1994). Making connections: towards an understanding of the role of networks in intersectoral collaboration for healthy public policy in cities. *Journal of Contemporary Health* (forthcoming).

Tsouros, A. (1991). *The healthy cities project: new developments and research needs*. Paper presented at a conference on Research for Healthy Cities, Glasgow, 1991.

UK Health for All Network (1993). *Health for All Resource Pack*. UKHFAN.

Walker, R. (1992). Interorganisational linkages for community health. *Health Promotion International*, 7(4), 257–264.

Webb, A. (1991). Coordination: a problem in public sector management. *Policy and Politics*, 19(4), 229–241.

Whetten, D. A. (1982). Objectives and issues: setting the stage. In D. L. Rogers & D. A. Whetten (eds), *op. cit.*

World Health Organisation (1984). *Health Promotion: A Discussion Document*. Copenhagen: WHO.

World Health Organisation (1985). *Targets for Health for All*. Copenhagen: WHO.

World Health Organisation (1986). *Ottawa Charter for Health Promotion. An International Conference on Health Promotion*, Nov 17–21. Geneva: WHO.

Zapka, J. G. *et al.* (1992). Inter-organisational responses to AIDS: a case study of the Worcester AIDS consortium. *Health Education Research: Theory and Practice*, 7(1), 31–46.

Health service

SECTION TWO

Health Science

3 The role of health authorities in the promotion of health

Lee Adams

Recently, the NHS has undergone another major restructuring, one of a long line of such changes; however, this last reorganisation has created fundamental new roles for health authorities at the same time as reforms affecting general practitioners and primary care.

The NHS reforms of 1990, by the Conservative government, have created what Ranude (1994) refers to as a quasi market, or managed competition; a structure of buyers and sellers caused by separating responsibility for the purchase of health care from its provision and allowing limited competition for business between providers.

Over the last few years, we have also seen changes to the way general practitioner (GP) services are organised, with the introduction of the model of purchasing by GPs who, under this scheme, became fundholders. The NHS now has two kinds of purchasers; health authorities and GPs. Furthermore, in 1996, health authorities and Family Health Services Authorities (FHSAs) will merge to create a single kind of health authority at a district level, and many are already working either jointly or in a merged way. At the time of writing, health authorities are working closely with GPs in various arrangements for purchasing purposes. It seems likely that if a Conservative government remains in office there will be a move for GPs to become total purchasers, purchasing nearly all services for their patients, and for the majority of GPs to be involved in purchasing in some form. This is likely to move quickly forward to a situation where health authorities' remaining roles are rather different from their current responsibilities.

In terms of Regional Health Authorities (RHAs), in 1994/95 these have been reorganised and reduced in number, becoming outposts of the NHS Executive. Within these changes, there is an overall move to reorientate the NHS to a primary care-led service. In an NHS Executive paper in late 1994 (NHS Executive, 1994) on this subject, it was stated that there would be a clear new role for health authorities to lead in developing and implementing a local health strategy, working in collaboration with GPs, NHS Trusts, local agencies and people, to develop a coherent view of health needs and the contributions the various parts of the NHS and local agencies can make towards meeting them.

If the Labour Party wins the next election, they are currently pledged to dismantle fundholding. However, whatever the outcome of the general election, it is generally believed that GPs will be a vital force in purchasing structures in the future.

What does all of this mean for health promotion?

The changes outlined above have had a profound effect on specialist health promotion services and, to a lesser extent, health promotion delivery by NHS providers. There has been a great debate in most District Health Authorities about where specialist services should be placed in terms of purchasing and providing (see also Chapter 6 of this volume for a discussion of the purchaser/provider split). This has led to enormous confusion and loss of morale (Society of Health Education and Promotion Specialists, 1993), as there has been no central guidance. Some health promotion specialist services (HPS) have been placed in providing Trusts while some have remained in purchasing authorities, though not all are involved in purchasing work, and some have had a split role and accountability. As health authorities struggled to come to terms with their new role, some specialist health promotion departments were moved first to providing and then, when the health authorities saw the error of their decision, back to purchasing.

All of this has been most unfortunate, and particularly ironic as in 1992 the government launched its national health promotion strategy *The Health of the Nation* (Department of Health, 1992). At the very time that health promotion was in ascendancy in the NHS and, indeed, nationally, in the rhetoric of government, the health promotion infrastructure in the NHS was being dismantled in many areas and thrown into disarray.

However, the new role of health authorities has had a number of positive and exciting implications for health promotion in terms of the role of health promotion specialists (see the next chapter for a further discussion of this), for the influence of a health promotion perspective and for the drawing up of strategies and activities to promote health.

The health promoting role of health authorities

Health authorities freed from having to manage provider services and, in time, free of most purchasing responsibilities, can now really come into their own as strategists for health improvements if they have the will and skills to do so.

One Minister for Health (Mawhinney, 1993) believed that purchasers should take the lead in forcing the pace of change. Their goal is to improve health and health services, and to change inappropriate ways of delivering clinical care and preventing illness.

There are various roles for health authorities in this scenario, which some have taken up vigorously while others have not, preferring to stick to a narrow view of purchasing as mainly contracting and managing the health services market and delivery. A health authority which sees a full public health role for itself could be engaging in the following kinds of activity:

- Health needs assessment/epidemiology;
- Contracting/purchasing with or on behalf of GPs;
- Research;
- Provider development;
- Strategic planning;
- Strategy development;
- Community development;
- Community participation;
- Public health advocacy;
- Campaigning/lobbying;
- Staff health development;
- Networking/healthy alliances;
- Quality assessment;
- Information development and provision:
    (i)   statutory
    (ii) provider assessment
    (iii) PHC information systems
    (iv) public information
- Public relations;
- Organisational development;
- Education and training – direct and by commission.

Health promotion and public health are not listed, but are implicit in all of the above. Health promotion specialists have particular skills and expertise to bring to many of the above functions (Society of Health Education and Promotion Specialists, 1994), as do public health specialists, and a combination of both is essential for a health authority to fulfil its role.

The aims of a health authority, it could be suggested, are threefold. Firstly, to develop health strategies involving providers and the public and other agencies; secondly, to secure accessible, appropriate and effective services for the public; and thirdly, to speak out to government and other local agencies on issues which are detrimental to health in their area (public health advocacy). This would be in order to promote well-being, reduce inequalities in health and reduce preventable death, illness and disability. The key to all of the above should be interagency partnerships and action, or healthy alliances.

Clearly, this new role of health authorities, together with the impetus of *The Health of the Nation* and the emphasis on health promotion within primary care and, indeed, the whole refocusing on primary care, provides many opportunities for health promotion influence and action. Within a health authority, health promotion can act through a variety of mechanisms and functions including: (a) within purchasing processes themselves; (b) among providers, and (c) via healthy alliances.

Health promotion within purchasing

Health promotion expertise is needed in all aspects of purchasing; for example, health promotion specialists need to be involved directly in purchasing and planning groups and subgroups, and involved in strategy development. The Sheffield health promotion specialists have been part of multidisciplinary strategic planning and purchasing groups, and from the beginning of the reforms, they have been able to bring a health promotion perspective as well as being directly responsible for health promotion aspects of the development and strategic work. In women's health, for example, planning and purchasing, HPS and public health doctors have together developed a strategy for women's health improvement with community participation and interagency liaison, and ensured input to other health strategies impacting upon women.

With the shift to more primary care-led purchasing, it is important to maintain a health promotion perspective, and much work will be needed with GPs and primary health care teams (PHCTs) to broaden horizons about what constitutes health promotion and to reorientate to a system of primary health care as opposed to the current primary medical care system.

Health promotion also has to be interwoven into quality specifications and monitoring. There are many areas of overlap; for example, the availability of health education information and a health promotion viewpoint can enrich quality development.

Within the contracting process, health promotion needs to be integrated into all mechanisms. Locally, in the Sheffield district, this has been achieved by:

1. Making it part of general requirements for all Trusts. It has been made explicit that health promotion is an important part of their

role and work, that principles of health promotion need to be adhered to and that the Trusts have a part to play in district-wide strategies for health improvement.

2. Ensuring that all service agreements, as appropriate, have a health promotion perspective and approach built in as well as specific health promotion objectives. For example, an accident and emergency specification to include accident prevention objectives.

3. All Trusts have had an appendix of health promotion requirements which sets the framework for activities, and specific overall objectives, for that year. This has shifted in time from being 'basic' requirements such as having a smoking policy in place, to now being linked to yearly themes, for example substance misuse, health promotion in the primary/secondary interface and health promotion linked to poverty issues.

4. Policy guidelines papers have been drawn up for Trusts as a guide to health authority policy implementation, to avoid all Trusts having to reinvent the wheel; these have been produced, for example, for sexual health, tobacco and alcohol.

5. An overall framework paper setting out what health promotion is and including principles was set out as a checklist in year 1 for the Trusts.

Health promotion among providers

All Trusts need mechanisms to coordinate their health promotion activity. Locally, for example, this has been achieved by a year 1 requirement for them all to designate a Health Promotion Link Person and set up a Health Promotion Coordinating Group. This has worked well and health promotion specialists in purchasing, support and advice link people as required, bringing them together for sharing, discussion and training. It is required that all link people in larger Trusts will acquire a health promotion qualification in a specific time frame. In addition, a senior health promotion specialist (Deputy Director), was seconded part-time for three months to one large Trust to assist in strategic development, once they had achieved a baseline of work. Again, this was useful experience for the health promotion specialist and invaluable high-level input for the Trust. This could be available to other Trusts if required.

Health promotion training is required and this is especially important if health promotion specialists are in purchasing, with, therefore, no infrastructure of health promotion expertise in providing Trusts; locally, one of the Universities developed a diploma/masters course in health promotion, and provided a health promotion seminar programme to support Trusts' health promotion work.

Health promotion via healthy alliances

The NHS is limited in what it can achieve for health improvement. *The Health of the Nation* legitimated healthy alliance work, though there was already much going on especially in northern cities in the UK before this. It is important that healthy alliances are strategic and based upon an agreement of principles, objectives and processes. In Sheffield, there is a well established Healthy City initiative, and there was a structure already developed which enabled links to purchasing work and the delivery of *The Health of the Nation* through a more broadly-based approach with the involvement of eight major partner agencies and a range of affiliate organisations in the city well-used to health promotion concepts and joint work (Healthy Sheffield, 1994a). In addition, the framework for health promotion drew on the Healthy City principles and local city health plan and the community development strategy to inform Trusts of requirements. Such structures and initiatives can assist purchasing in many ways and clarify the particular part the NHS has to play in improving health locally.

Other approaches

In addition to the above, health promotion can be developed from purchasing in the organisation of health promotion programmes targeted at:

(a) Population groups, such as children and young people;
(b) Health issues, for example tobacco;
(c) Prerequisites for health, for example concerning poverty or housing;
(d) A geographic area in the district.

These can be led by purchasers working closely with Trusts, voluntary organisations and statutory and commercial bodies. Pilot or demonstration projects also have a useful role to play in trial approaches and in demonstrating lessons for duplication elsewhere; projects will sometimes be run as part of purchasing itself, via PHC teams, or by commissioning a project.

Constraints and dilemmas

A major constraint in all of this can be how health authorities view health promotion. Health promotion is sometimes seen quite narrowly from a medical model perspective, and, understandably, health authorities have often embraced *The Health of the Nation* as a set of targets, without fully taking on board the Health for All philosophy.

Health promotion is made up of many different disciplines applied to health in a positive way; practitioners and theoreticians often take a social model as a framework and draw on the Health for All principles of equity, participation and intersectoral partnerships. Health promotion also asserts that work is required on the prerequisites for health (Adams and Pintus, 1994).

Although it embraces some aspects of Health for All, *The Health of the Nation* does, unfortunately, focus on an individual behaviour change approach. A useful critique of *The Health of the Nation* and a comparison with public health strategies in one city initiative (Thomas, 1993), shows that there are differences in the way health is defined, the way in which determinants of health are understood and the different disciplinary bases of these strategies. The study concludes that the strategies stand at the opposite ends of the spectrum of current thinking and approaches in public health, with the WHO strategy falling somewhere in between, though closer to the city perspective. Health authorities have to adhere to and deliver national strategies. However, they will also have to develop their own local strategies based on need and on a local perspective. It could be argued that health promotion expertise is vital to these processes, which will need to include the five tenets of the Ottawa Charter (WHO, 1986) building healthy public policy, creating supportive environments, strengthening community action, developing personal skills and reorienting health services.

Health authorities will, if they want to really improve health and reduce inequalities as opposed to adopting a narrow approach to health gain (Adams, 1994), need to work in a dynamic way which recognises that to promote health will require focusing on economic, social and environmental policy.

A helpful rhetoric to emerge with the NHS reforms has been that of community involvement, and there have been a series of guidance statements emphasising that health authorities need to involve local people in policy and planning. This is another opportunity for health promotion in that participation is a key principle, and also that health promotion specialists form one of the few NHS disciplines to have expertise in this area. Many health authorities have developed mechanisms to consult with local people; however, few have formal mechanisms in place to involve people in decision making. Furthermore, to really involve people would require processes of community development to underpin participation strategies and enable local people to become involved. There are encouraging signs that community development may be gaining credence with purchasers; some have employed community development workers and many are purchasing community development programmes. However, there are dilemmas and contradictions for health authorities here. The reforms have made health authorities less democratic in the composition of boards, not more so, and also I wonder as health authorities really start to involve people in expressing needs and having a say in decisions, if this will be welcomed by government, as such processes tend to lead to people expressing basic needs concerned with housing, poverty and environmental issues (Healthy Sheffield, 1994). Issues of poverty are absent from *The Health of the Nation*. This aside, a move towards community development approaches to health promotion, which can be health promoting in themselves, and as an enablement to participation, holds a lot of hope for effective purchasing. As purchasing shifts to GPs, this area of work will have to be reinforced and linked more to the PHC setting.

Finally, a major constraint and dilemma will be how far health authorities will feel able to act as champions of the people's health. Health authorities have been known to lobby government about such issues as tobacco taxation; whether health authorities will lobby government with regard to such fundamental issues as pollution, remains to be seen, and how far they feel able to lobby local government, often a healthy alliance partner, over their policies, will also be an area of difficulty requiring political skill and judgement. Nevertheless, as we do not have overt voices at present speaking out for the public's health, health authorities, together with local people and other agencies, could be a powerful force for possible action and change.

At present, it seems likely that health authorities who have a role in planning, policy development and strategy can play a key role in drawing together partnerships through their own fields of influence, and, in combination with GPs, in promoting health.

It needs to be acknowledged that health authorities and the NHS are limited in what they can directly achieve, and the political role a health authority can play in negotiating, networking and lobbying will be vital. This will call for skills which health authorities need to ensure they have on board or are able to develop. This role will call for a broadly-based definition of health promotion which is based upon a social model of health and a health promotion strategy which attempts to meet locally defined need – including prerequisites for health and the reduction of inequalities.

Health authorities will need to carve space for themselves in this role, to deliver national priorities but also to focus on locally expressed need. There may be contradictions here, to be negotiated.

Health authorities need to develop an approach to health promotion that is based more on Health for All approaches and principles, including reorienting services to primary health care; they will need to develop secondary and tertiary services to maximise their health promotion potential.

Health authorities will need to realise that their role needs to focus on health improvement. For many, this will be a considerable shift in focus from primarily managing and then commissioning illness and care services. It is vital that health authorities have the expertise needed to fulfil this new role.

References

Adams, L. (1994). Response – health promotion in crisis. *Health Education Journal*, 53, 345–360.

Adams, L. & Pintus, S. (1994). A challenge to prevailing theory and practice. *Critical Public Health*, 5(2), 17–29.

Department of Health (1992). *The Health of the Nation*. London: HMSO.

Healthy Sheffield (1994a). A range of Healthy Sheffield documents detailing its work are available from the Healthy Sheffield Development Unit, Town Hall Chambers, 1 Barkers Pool, Sheffield, S1 1EN.

Healthy Sheffield (1994b). *Our City, Our Health – What You Said. Ibid.*

Mawhinney, B. (1993). Speech to the Association for Public Health Annual Conference, Chester: APH.

NHS Management Executive (1994). *Developing NHS Purchasing and GP Fundholding. Towards a Primary Care Led NHS*. NHSME.

Ranude, W. (1994). *A Future for the NHS?* London: Longman.

Society of Health Education and Promotion Specialists (1993). *Health Promotion At The Crossroads: A Study of Health Promotion Departments in the reorganised NHS*. SHEPS.

Society of Health Education and Promotion Specialists (1994). *The Role of the Health Promotion Specialist in the NHS*. SHEPS.

Thomas, C. (1993). Public health strategies in Sheffield and England – A comparison of conceptual foundations. *Health Promotion International*, 8(4), 299–307.

World Health Organisation (1986). *Ottawa Charter for Health Promotion*. Geneva: WHO.

4 The role of the Family Health Services Authorities in promoting health

Penny Astrop and Jonathan McWilliam

To understand the influence of Family Health Service Authorities (FHSAs) on health promotion, it is helpful to understand what an FHSA does. At the time of writing, the British Government is preparing legislation which will merge FHSAs and District Health Authorities to form a new type of health authority comprising the functions of both its predecessors. The new authorities are likely to be established in 1996. The details of their structure and function remain unspecified. It is, however, reasonable to assume that the present functions of FHSAs will continue within the new bodies, especially since the centrally negotiated contracts of general practitioners (GPs), dentists, pharmacists and opticians remain in place.

Prior to the NHS reforms of 1990, it was the duty of Family Practitioner Committees (FPCs) to administer the contracts of GPs, general dental practitioners, community pharmacists and opticians. These family practitioners were, and still are, independent contractors and are not employees of the NHS. In 1989 the FPCs were replaced by Family Health Service Authorities. The new authorities still retained the duty described above but, importantly, they were given greater freedom and responsibility for local implementation of the nationally negotiated contract in order to provide family health services for the given population. As a consequence, the FHSA is also concerned with the access to and quality of those services.

There are currently approximately 90 FHSAs in England, serving populations ranging from about 130 000 to 1 600 000. Each FHSA conforms to a major local authority area and increasingly they match the geographical boundaries of District Health Authorities, as they in turn are reshaped. FHSAs are accountable to Regional Health Authorities, which are also undergoing change at the time of writing.

FHSAs perform a number of functions, which include:

- Administering and approving applications by practitioners to enter into contract or vary their terms and conditions;

- Maintaining the national GP registration data base and arranging the transfer of medical records;
- Managing primary care development funds;
- Paying practitioners in accordance with the national statement of fees and allowances (the Red Book);
- Providing information to the public;
- Dealing with complaints made by patients;
- Introducing medical audit;
- Monitoring and improving GP prescribing;
- Approving surgery locations and hours of availability.

More recently, FHSAs have been involved, with the regions, to recruit, develop and monitor GP fundholders. The impact of GP fundholding has been significant throughout the whole of the NHS, and with the changes in regional structure more responsibility for this will fall on the new health authorities. In the meantime, in areas where fundholding is popular, it represents a major workload for the FHSA.

The FHSA does work most frequently with GPs, but involvement with dentists and pharmacists is important. However, the absence of many actual powers or inducements to influence dentists or pharmacists tends to make the relationship more of a paper exercise.

Relationships with optical services are minimal in most FHSAs, restricted mainly to purely administrative tasks. This reflects the reducing amount of work done by these practitioners within the NHS.

In order to influence the quality of services, leading-edge FHSAs also tend to be involved in local, non-statutory initiatives, often in association with other groups such as continuing-medical-education tutors and nurse trainers. These often provide direct training and support to practitioners and their staff.

The FHSAs' position in the wider NHS

FHSAs have formal relationships, as described above, with Regional Health Authorities and family practitioners. They also have links with many other bodies, and work particularly closely with District Health Authorities and local representative committees of GPs, dentists, pharmacists and opticians. Relationships with social services departments are becoming increasingly important following community care legislation. Links with consumer bodies such as the Community Health Council and voluntary agencies are frequent. Closer relationships between Family Health Services Authorities, District Health Authorities and social services departments mean that planning and managing health and social care as an integrated whole becomes a more attainable goal. This should help to create better integrated health promotion services.

The statutory contribution of FHSAs to health promotion

General practice

The contribution of GPs has been dealt with elsewhere in this book and will not be greatly expanded further here. However, it is important to note that with the revised 1990 GP contract, the terms of service for the first time required GPs to give appropriate advice to patients with regard to health and specific lifestyle activities, such as smoking. This was significant as up until this time a GP had no stated responsibilities in health promotion.

This responsibility is over and above the special banded payments they can receive for carrying out health promotion programmes. As with all such special allowances, the FHSA must first approve its payment and in applying for an allowance the GP will submit a description of how the health programmes will be carried out. In order to monitor progress and compliance, anonymised data relating to the programmes is submitted to the FHSA, on an annual basis. This data can be aggregated and fed back to GPs in a comparative format. This can then be used as a planning tool for FHSA and GP alike, and this is covered in more detail below.

Dentists

The basis of the 1990 contract with general dental practitioners was to move away from a payment system based on active treatment to one that encouraged registration of patients and rewarded dentists for providing preventive treatment and advice , especially to children. The spirit of the new contract was welcomed by the profession as well as dental health promoters. However, the intention of the new contract was never realised because the profession failed to agree with the government on the accompanying financial settlement. In areas where practice expenses were high, particularly in south-east England, this has led to significant withdrawal of dentists from the NHS. At the time of writing, the publication of a new White Paper covering reforms of NHS dental treatment is awaited. The government did publish a long awaited Oral Health Strategy in 1994 (Department of Health, 1994) but this was dependent in part on stable service provision within the NHS.

The FHSA has always had less statutory powers with regard to dentistry, than it has with GPs. Dentists in contract with the NHS are able to mix their NHS work with private work and are not obliged to accept patients for NHS treatment. Only if they fail to do any NHS work in six months does their contract with the NHS automatically lapse. The patient registration and practitioner payments are processed by a separate body, the Dental Practice Board. However, in parts of the country less effected by high practice expenses, there still remains a substantial NHS service. FHSAs in these areas are more likely to be involved in the development of non-statutory services and health promotion campaigns. For example, some have encouraged registration with a dentist by placing information in medical record cards as part of a locally targeted dental health promotion campaign.

Pharmacists

The FHSA has a complex and quasi-judicial role in granting approval for the opening of a new chemist's shop or granting approval for a GP to start dispensing medicines from a practice. This is governed by a detailed set of statutory guidance, and all decisions are subject to appeal to the Secretary of State. In considering such applications, the FHSA will need to consider what access a population has to pharmaceutical services, and these increasingly include health promotion and advice from pharmacists and their staff. In 1993, FHSAs were granted powers to make special payments to pharmacists for providing such advice in accordance with agreed local standards. This extends the role of the pharmacist and makes them an increasingly significant member of the wider primary health care team (PHCT).

Opticians

As has already been stated, the FHSAs statutory involvement with opticians is minimal, as very little of their total work is carried out under the NHS. The quality of service is governed by the profession. The FHSAs do process claims for exemption from NHS fees by certain restricted groups, such as people with diabetes. This has in turn led to some FHSAs working with local opticians, DHAs and specialists to develop screening services for at-risk groups at local level.

The specific non-statutory influence of FHSAs

FHSAs have considerable discretion over their own way of working once they step outside their statutory obligations. Some examples of the types of influence an FHSA can bring to bear on health promotion are described below.

Developing the primary health care team as a health promoting organisation

Many FHSAs have developed the concept of the Primary Care Facilitator first described by the Oxford Prevention of Heart Attack and Stroke Project (Fullard *et al.*, 1987) to suit their own needs. Not all FHSAs will employ facilitators as such, but all will have some staff working on service and/or quality development who will be using a facilitative style of working, because experience has shown that it is the most appropriate way to work with independent contractors. FHSAs who adopted a top-heavy management or policing style of service development in the early days quickly learned the error of their ways as GPs simply exercised their right to work strictly to the terms of service and the rules contained within the Red Book, thus stifling any FHSA innovation.

The primary care facilitators, before the 1990 GP contract, worked by persuading GPs that health promotion activities should and could be on the primary health care agenda. They often did this by encouraging and developing the role of other members of the team most notably the practice nurse (Astrop, 1988). The 1990 contract, as has already been mentioned, firmly put health promotion on the agenda for primary care. This enabled facilitators to spend less time *selling* the health promotion idea and more time helping GPs deliver it.

The concept of the whole PHCT as a health promoting body was not a new one, but the practical barriers to team working make it difficult for some to achieve. Facilitators began to concentrate on helping teams to work together, recognising their complementary roles as well as the team opportunities to promote health.

Facilitation is at its heart a practical and pragmatic approach to getting professionals to change their practice. As such, a facilitator has to walk a fine line between achieving the objectives of the FHSA and the wider NHS, and meeting the presenting needs of the PHCT with whom they are working. As well as specific teaching, management and communication skills, facilitators will use a variety of strategies, from the production of written guidelines to the organisation of team away-days and training events. Each FHSA will have its own style and quality of relationship with its practitioners, and this will in turn influence what its service development staff do. Some FHSAs are reducing the number of staff they employ directly to do this kind of work, and are devolving development monies (and in some cases staff budgets) to the teams so that they can buy in the services of outside consultants as required.

This in turn requires an increasingly sophisticated level of practice management than was previously the case. Fundholding has also influenced the pace of development of practice management. Many FHSAs now see their most important role in support of primary health care to be assisting in the development of high quality general management of primary health care teams. For example, the 1990 contract required GPs to produce an annual report. On the whole this is a fairly sterile exercise, but it can be used as a hook on which to hang the introduction of the concept of planning to primary health care teams. In this context it is necessary for the whole team to consider the total health needs of their population. Once they do this they will begin to tackle not only the way they as individuals can promote the health of patients, but also how they can promote the health of the whole population as a team. This will encourage them to see themselves as one of many influencers on health in the community. The importance of working with others such as schools, voluntary groups and local business starts to become a natural step. In the past, general practice could be characterised as being isolated and almost totally reactive in the way it provided care. Encouraging planning immediately makes it necessary for the GP to look around for the causes of ill health and seek the help of others both in the immediate team and in the wider community.

Those who have already begun this approach are benefiting from the feeling of the team taking more control of their work load and being able to argue constructively for more resources. FHSAs concerned with low morale amongst GPs can use this kind of development to counteract the sense of contributory disempowerment. Fundholding has had a similar effect and indeed it is the fundholding GPs who often lead the way in the development of strategic planning.

By creating similar opportunities for non-fundholding GPs, FHSAs can ensure that all patients feel the benefits of being served by a health promoting primary health care team.

Encouraging health promotion through ongoing FHSA activities

FHSAs can choose to inject an element of health promotion in many of their ongoing functions. The FHSA has a responsibility to inform the public how they can access the various family practitioner services. Some FHSAs take this a step further by including health promotion messages in routine information that is sent to all patients. Under the Patient's Charter initiative, FHSAs are trying to raise their own profile with the public and some have developed high-street offices where members of the public can get information about health and related services. This is often supplemented with more direct health promotion information. Other FHSAs have established patient helplines or more proactive relationships with local media, often becoming involved in local events such as health fairs.

The FHSA may work with its local Medical Audit Advisory Group to encourage GPs to undertake audits of their health promotion activity and identify ways in which it could be improved. The various initiatives FHSAs have developed to influence cost-effective prescribing often have a health promotion effect. For example, a practice reviewing the use of psychotropic drugs may review the potential role of a counsellor to offer alternative treatments for the promotion of mental health. Several FHSAs have been instrumental in developing *prescription for exercise* schemes (in partnership with GPs and local authorities).

The non-statutory influence of FHSAs on other practitioner groups

Some FHSAs have commissioned local health promotion campaigns. For example, in dental health promotion campaigns as previously mentioned, or campaigns encouraging the disposal of unwanted medicines to promote the prevention of accidents. In working with pharmacists, the introduction of needle exchange schemes has been at the forefront of influencing safe practice amongst intravenous drug users.

As independent practitioners, GPs and dentists are employers in their own right and, as such, responsibility under health and safety legislation is entirely theirs. FHSAs often develop an advisory and information service to help them in this area. An example of how this influences health promotion would be ensuring dentists and doctors have up-to-date information on the latest standards in the sterilisation of instruments. In order to encourage practitioners to buy necessary new equipment to meet standards, some FHSAs go further to help. For instance, bulk purchase of more expensive equipment may be arranged to gain discounts for individual practices.

The wider influence of FHSAs in health promotion

Links to district health authorities and departments of public health medicine

The NHS Executive requires FHSAs to work with District Health Authorities on many items of health policy. Arrangements are also made for FHSAs to receive public health advice. Both of these routes allow two-way influence to be exerted. A specific example of this would be joint working on primary health care team development which would coordinate activity between general practitioners and practice-employed staff on the one hand and health visitors and district nurses on the other hand. This is a useful way of strengthening the health promotion role of health visitors within the primary health care team.

A further example is the encouragement of a health promoting dental service by coordinating the integration of NHS dentists with District Health Authority policies on fluoridation, referral to oral-surgery departments, use of X-ray equipment and arrangements for emergency dental care.

As the merger with District Health Authorities approaches, it is becoming second nature for FHSAs and DHAs to make policy decisions together. This can mean working to develop strategies across primary and secondary care covering both specific conditions such as coronary heart disease, and care groups such as care of the elderly. This allows an integration of strategies for health promotion, so that a joint approach can be taken to coronary heart disease to cover health promotion and primary, secondary and tertiary prevention of disease. These links have been strengthened by *The Health of the Nation* initiative (Department of Health, 1992) which specifies that a joint approach is necessary.

Joint policy work of this kind can also be carried out with both District Health Authorities and social services departments, particularly for specific care groups. This allows exciting developments such as coordinated approaches to improving child health, bringing together immunisation campaigns, the role of the health visitor in schools and prevention and early detection of child abuse.

The FHSA also has an opportunity to *manage up* through its managerial relationship to Regional Health Authorities. There is little doubt that the concerted efforts of a number of FHSAs influenced the amendments to the health promotion arrangements originally set out in the 1990 GP contract. As these arrangements originally appeared, they actually made it more difficult for teams to adopt an integrated, opportunistic approach. The new banding system reflected more appropriately the best models of practice developed by teams and also allowed FHSAs potentially to make meaningful use of the monitoring data the practices are required to collect.

Developmental roles for FHSAs

Leading edge FHSAs can use their discretion to develop their role. Examples of this are, development of localities and the development of an equal-opportunities culture in all health care.

Locality development is often focused on secondary care being purchased by local people including GPs, as a kind of alternative to fundholding. FHSAs are concerned primarily with influencing primary and community care provision; therefore when they become involved in locality development, they tend to emphasise other equally important aspects of locality development, such as encouraging local providers of health and social care to work together to provide a more seamless service based around the local surgeries. Another example is to engage local people in the planning and purchasing of local services.

Equal opportunity of access to health care has long been neglected by health authorities. However, some FHSAs have done pioneering work in developing primary care services with specific populations in mind. For example, homeless people, those from minority ethnic groups and young people.

Others have carried out work with existing primary health care teams to improve services. Most notably, work has been undertaken to encourage the employment of female GPs in practices, and to raise awareness of the specific health promotion needs of people from different ethnic groups.

In the future, the existence of a new combined health authority will create new opportunities for health promotion. FHSAs are already beginning to work on forward planning in primary health care, and this could lead in due course to local contracts between primary health care teams and the new health authorities. This could increase the ability of new health authorities to strengthen health promotion in primary health care teams.

The future of dental health care hangs in the balance. Health authorities will have to decide, with a reduced service commitment, where priorities lie. Dental health promotion will become an important issue and may become a major priority if levels of dental health in the population fall.

The real challenge for the new health authorities will be to develop a health service, as opposed to an ill-health service, and to integrate this into a wider community whilst strengthening patient choice. People will need better information and clearer messages about health promotion from health professionals. This all requires major shifts in knowledge and attitudes of the health providers and purchasers of the future.

References

Astrop, P. J. (1988). What the facilitator can do for the practice nurse. *Practice Nurse*, May 1988.

Department of Health (1992.) *The Health of the Nation: A Strategy for Health in England.* London: HMSO.

Department of Health (1994). *An Oral Health Strategy for England.* London: HMSO.

Fullard, E., Fowler, G. & Gray, M. (1987). Promoting prevention in primary care: controlled trial of low technology, low cost approach. *British Medical Journal, 294,* 1080–2.

5 Health promotion in primary health care

Judy Orme and Cheryl Wright

Health promotion over the last 20 years has been given increased emphasis in the primary health care setting. Tannahill (1988) suggests that primary health care and health promotion may be seen as twin pillars of the *Health for All by the Year 2000* strategy (World Health Organisation, 1985).

The problematical development of a symbiotic relationship between health promotion and primary health care (PHC) is central to this chapter. Problematical in the sense that a holistic model of health is the epistemological base to health promotion; but the dominant interpretation of primary health care in this country is based on a medical orientation to health. The dilemmas for general practice that this produces are discussed along with the opportunities for health promotion. The health visitor is selected for particular scrutiny, as an example of how the role of PHC professions in health promotion may be supported and sustained.

The delivery of health promotion in general practice

The origin of this increased focus on health promotion in primary health care stems from the unique access which general practitioners (GPs) have to the population (Williams *et al.*, 1993). Over 95 per cent of the population are registered with a GP and on average consult a doctor four times a year. Changes in the structure of delivery of health promotion in primary care since the introduction of the 1990 GP contract have been very rapid and health promotion is now enshrined in the duties of every GP (Department of Health, 1989a). GPs are currently working in areas of data collection, audit and health promotion which they have not necessarily been trained to do. With the introduction of the 1990 GP contract and its subsequent revisions, the focus on health promotion in PHC could be argued to have become increasingly narrow due to the emphasis put on remuneration linked to specific objectives.

The original contract encouraged practices to introduce health promotion clinics by offering a sessional fee for each clinic. In response to alleged abuse of the clinic-based system, where practices could run any number of clinics and be paid for them, a moratorium on starting new clinics was introduced in June 1993. However, the legacy of this clinic-based system is likely to have emphasised the manageability of a compartmentalised lifestyles approach to health promotion for both the GP and the patient.

Payments for health promotion clinics changed to new banding arrangements in July 1993. These combine opportunistic work with a banding system (band 1 is the lowest and band 3 the highest) linked to objectives in *The Health of the Nation* (Department of Health, 1992) to reduce smoking, coronary heart disease and strokes. There is also separate recognition and payment for organised programmes of care to help people manage their diabetes and asthma. Over 90 per cent of GPs were approved to run programmes in band 3 (Department of Health, 1993c).

The speed with which these changes have been imposed, and the nature of these changes have contributed to a lowered morale amongst general practitioners, where job satisfaction is low and levels of anger and cynicism are high (Calnan *et al.*, 1994; Orme, 1994). In a recent survey of GPs in Great Britain (General Service Medical Committee, 1992) more than 82 per cent of respondents agreed that, 'too much is being asked of general practice at the present time'. It is important to see this lowered morale as a backcloth to the present changes in health promotion and to acknowledge the influence this may have on future health promotion within general practice.

Anger and cynicism amongst GPs towards the changes in delivery of health promotion has been fuelled by several factors. These include, firstly, the perceived lack of Government commitment to tackling the underlying inequalities in health. Secondly, the introduction of payment for health promotion is seen by some GPs as an imposition on their work and professional autonomy (Orme, 1994). There is continued debate about the effectiveness of health promotion (Stott *et al.*, 1994; Imperial Cancer Research Fund OXCHECK Study Group 1994; Family Heart Study Group, 1994; Cupples and McKnight, 1994). Within a market economy, the evaluation of health promotion initiatives is being encouraged in terms of outcomes and not processes (Ewles, 1995) and yet maximum benefit would be gained by involving both. Thirdly, significant perceived barriers to health promotion have been identified by GPs which include time, resources, workload, stress and exhaustion (Kaufman, 1990).

Promoting health in areas of deprivation

Stott *et al.* (1994) question the value of a blanket approach to lifestyle change in PHC without a supportive environment. Difficulties are particularly apparent when working with a clinic-based system in deprived areas (Main and Main, 1990). Evidence suggests that the inverse care law (Tudor Hart, 1971) applies with health promotion clinics and also to invitations to health checks. Those people in most need do not attend. Primary health care teams (PHCTs) working with these communities need to be given opportunities to have their voices heard to facilitate appropriate supportive strategies being developed.

The new GP contract did provide extra remuneration (deprivation allowance) for practices in areas of high deprivation (Jarman, 1983), but the payments continue to be based on 1981 census data rather than the 1991 figures. It is estimated that there has been a 10 per cent increase in the number of residents in deprived wards of cities over the interim ten years (Brown, 1995). Also, the Jarman index upon which decisions about deprivation allowances are made, is a composite score based on whole electoral wards and consequently localities of deprivation and high need are often invisible next to more affluent areas which alter the Jarman score. Unemployment rates (Campbell *et al.*, 1991) and long-standing illness would be more appropriate indicators of population health needs. With the merging of District Health Authorities and FHSAs there is increased potential to focus on felt and expressed needs of smaller defined localities. It is officially recognised that GPs working in deprived areas need help in coping with deprivation and its implications for health (Royal College of General Practitioners, 1991; Craft and Dillner, 1994). This indisputable evidence urgently needs to be translated into appropriate resourcing.

Potential within the consultation

The GP consultation remains at the heart of PHC albeit with the many added external pressures (Stott, 1993). These pressures include national targets, accounting, management and organisation within the PHCT, and charters increasing the pressure from consumerism. The varying impact of these pressures may be acting as distractions from the consultation process, but may also be seen as creating opportunities for health promotion. It is this covert potential that must be recognised and prioritised.

Stott (1993) believes there is exceptional potential within every consultation in primary care. This potential he divides into four areas, the management of presenting problems and of continuing problems, modification of help-seeking behaviour and opportunistic health promotion. The latter two categories are the important sections for the future development of appropriate but innovative health promotion. Stott suggests that there is potential for problems presented in the consultation to be considered in the socioeconomic context of people's lives, and appropriate strategies for help encouraged. This process of 'modification of help-seeking behaviour' by GPs is important in facilitating the process of self-empowerment of patients. Integrating individual models of behaviour change in this way with a community development approach using community-based networks is sound underpinning for effective health promotion (Dowell and Gosling, 1993). Most GPs see their role in prevention to be in opportunistic health promotion and when used in context this is likely to be very effective. One of the dilemmas for the GP now is having to give lifestyle advice which is unrelated to the original reason for consultation (Daykin *et al.*, 1995).

Potential for health promotion within the banding arrangements

Health Promotion is an increasingly complex field, and to facilitate effective health promotion within a PHC setting demands a multifaceted approach including all the primary health care team (PHCT) together with community groups and organisations. Downie *et al.* (1992) believe that effective health promotion requires alliances between many different agencies including health authorities, social services and the voluntary sector. However, as Hanlon *et al.* (1990) suggest, collaborative approaches were not facilitated by the clinic and target-based system of payment.

The 1993 banding arrangements, however, encourage 'working with other individuals and agencies'. The reality of this potential depends on how this phrase from the banding documents is being interpreted in PHC. The official interpretation is, 'Work jointly when appropriate with other individuals or agencies to further the aims of the programme' (Department of Health, 1993a). There is evidence to suggest that some interpretations of 'working with other individuals and agencies' may be 'having other people to help do the work' (Orme, 1994). *The Health of the Nation* promotes the establishment and strengthening of 'Healthy Alliances'. The Department of Health's list of essential components for healthy alliances is formidable; a shared vision, common agendas, agreed priorities, openness about self-interest, mutual respect, trust, ability to learn from others and cultural sensitivity (Department of Health, 1993b). These features, however, mask a host of potential problems, which include possible conflicts, abrasive relationships, mutual recriminations, incompatible priorities, a lack of resources and little genuine commitment to either the process or aims of joint working. A more realistic list would include generosity of time and effort, initiative, generous personalities, open forums, community links and many other qualities. How can these be supported and encouraged in the pressured milieu of general practice?

Examples of good practice

Effective sharing of existing examples of good practice needs to be expanded to encompass the increasing number of initiatives where PHCTs work collaboratively towards health gain. These include: prescription for exercise initiatives (Biddle *et al.*, 1994; Jelley, 1993; Stockport Health Authority, 1993; Ireland, 1995); community development projects (Royal College of General Practitioners, 1994); and practice-based initiatives, for example welfare advice (Paris and Player, 1993), counselling and alternative therapists. Fundholding practices, in particular, are starting to employ complementary therapists (Naidoo and Wills, 1994). The impact of GP fundholding is discussed in Chapter 3 of this book.

Multi-layered communication is essential within the PHCT itself, between the PHCT and patients and between the practice and its community. The level of communication within the PHCT needs to be high so that a team approach to planning health promotion strategies is facilitated. This is being prioritised by a major workshop programme for members of the PHCT (Health Education Authority, 1991).

The role of health visitors in health promotion

The integration of practice nurses, district nurses, health visitors and other community nurses into the PHCT and a mutual understanding of their roles in health promotion, is vital to effectively promote health. In a recent study (Calnan *et al.*, 1994) it was found that arrangements in general practice tended to encourage health promotion which revolved around the practice nurse and which hindered the development of a broader team-based approach to the delivery of appropriate health promotion. Health visitors and district nurses were found to have a low level of involvement in practice-based clinic health promotion activity.

Community-based professionals such as health visitors, however, are in the forefront of recent government and World Health Organisation initiatives that promote healthy lifestyles in the general public (Department of Health, 1992; World Health Organisation, 1986).

Further consideration will now be given to the unique role of the health visitor and the potential within that role for health promotion.

Health promotion is an integral part of the health visiting service. Strategies which attempt to go beyond the individualistic model to address the full range of factors giving rise to ill-health in the wider community require collaboration between different health and welfare professions. However, Prentice (1991) argues that interprofessional cooperation and teamworking is becoming increasingly strained as services to clients become fragmented between provider groups. In the new enterprise culture of the NHS, there is pressure on health visitors to be proactive and to show that the skills they have to offer are cost-effective, and above all marketable. Health visitors also need to ensure that the contracts made with purchasers include objectives of their own and it must be recognised that effective measures of health promotion require agendas to be set in a collaborative way with the groups with whom the health visitor interacts (Health Visitors' Association, 1994; Pearson *et al.*, 1993).

Assessment of need

Health visitors are able to target the health needs of a given client population, using effective health profiling techniques whilst taking into account social factors such as housing, poverty and the needs of ethnic minority communities. This kind of research-based information should be used in business plans and specifications as part of the contract in order to relate service provision to identified health need, and to show how a particular pattern of resource allocation and skill mix is responding to it. The banding arrangements in PHC highlight the identification of *priority groups* which also provides scope for the development of targeted health promotion programmes within a practice population. The role of FHSAs in supporting and encouraging this process is critical and is discussed in the preceding chapter.

Advocacy for health

People do not experience health, social and financial problems, as separate problems and it is not helpful to them when agencies respond to them as such. Health visitors can act as advocates for people living in poverty, helping them to negotiate access to services. It is important to work towards transferring knowledge and skills to local people so that they can have the information and resources to challenge the social and economic causes of poverty themselves (Golding, 1986; Garmston, 1994; French, 1990). This approach reflects the self-empowerment model of health promotion interpreted in a community setting as advocated by the Ottawa Charter (World Health Organisation, 1986).

Health profiling can provide a framework from which inter-agency collaboration and community participation can be directed (Cernik and Wearne, 1991). It provides a basis from which a collective and negotiated response to health needs can be formulated and in which the community can take an active part. By targeting, the health visiting service can enable individuals and communities to make informed choices which may lead to an increased effectiveness in the use of current health care services and a decrease in the incidence of health-damaging behaviour and related morbidity and mortality.

The integration of these skills with those of mediation, enablement and advocacy at a local and intersectoral level allows a truly proactive approach to health promotion. Health visitors are in a prime position to influence health authority purchasing strategies, and thus the development of services and their skills are invaluable to purchasers of local health services. Several government documents provide a policy framework within which the contracts for health visiting services should be drawn up, governing both the range and quality of services to be commissioned. These include their influence on health care provision through multi-agency collaboration (Tomlinson, 1992; Department of Health, 1989b, 1991; Moores, 1993). These documents make a clear case for the need for qualified, skilled health visitors and school nurses to take forward the government's strategy for the future development of NHS services.

Health visitors are under increasing pressure from managers to evaluate their work, most commonly being presented with methods which refer only to numbers, costs and time taken. These systems often have less to do with the quality of service than with the need to cut costs and give managers simple indicators with which to bargain for resources. However, measuring the quality of the service is more complex than those systems allow (Black and Townsend, 1982).

Public health approaches within a market economy

There is a consensus of opinion which argues that although the new contract culture opens the way for diversity and innovation, health is not a commodity which can be bought and sold in packages as it is deeply rooted in the socioeconomic, gender and racial context in which the individual lives (Naish and Kline, 1990; Labour Party, 1990; Brent Community Health Council, 1981; Hunter, 1993; Williams *et al.*, 1993; Carr-Hill *et al.*, 1989; Moores *et al.*, 1993). There are advantages, nevertheless, resulting from the NHS reforms. For example, in working more closely with the newly formed Health Commissions, access to information about the health and characteristics of local practice populations has improved, and is useful to health visitors in identifying priorities for intervention and as a source of political pressure to increase resources for those client groups most in need (Acheson, 1988). Moores *et al.* (1993) underline the importance of multi-sectoral collaboration with regard to the public health aspect of primary care nursing. However, Orr (1991) argues that multi-agency working is now complicated by contractual relationships between some of the partners. Pearson (1993) argues that users themselves must be involved in service planning to avoid services becoming less accessible.

Several inherent difficulties in reconciling public health approaches within a market-led health care system have been illustrated leading to a potential decrease in collaboration and public accountability (Klein, 1992; Orr, 1991). Both Orr and Klein argue that the recent changes in the NHS may also make community participation and development difficult due to short-term goals, and contracts where long-term ideas of participation may have low priority. The need is also recognised for 'safety net' community nursing services for people not registered with a GP, such as the homeless and travellers, those who prefer to use neighbourhood or local services such as 'drop-in' centres and hospital accident and emergency departments. A blueprint of how general practice can address the needs of such groups and take on the wider issues of health promotion from a public health perspective is provided by Moores *et al.* (1993). The new public health demands a much broader vision of purchasing for health gain and is an issue high on the health service agenda (Watkins, 1991).

More recently, the separation between purchasing and providing health care has emphasised the responsibility of purchasers to assess the health needs of their populations. Purchasers are evaluating the extent to which health care providers are meeting those needs and improving health. Publication of targets for health, like those in *The Health of the Nation* White Paper, gives a framework for both purchasers and providers to achieve health improvements in the population. PHCT professionals who witness the effects of poverty and the wider environment on the health of individuals and families on a daily basis, therefore have much to contribute towards the new public health movement.

Recent, radical changes in the Health Service have encouraged PHCTs to conduct a re-examination of the service they have to offer. In the current climate, the PHCT needs to be able to effectively target their work towards specific client groups. Also, the challenge of current health trends demonstrates the need to provide a new public health service which is both consumer led and meets the demands for a high-quality, cost-effective, enterprise-efficient service. Key players in this are GPs and health visitors. The opportunities for health promotion within the consultation, through other practice-based initiatives and through collaborative working within community networks need prioritising.

Within the community, people enjoy universal access to health visitors, with no stigma attached. There are therefore important benefits to be derived by the local community and purchasers from the effective use of health visitors particularly with regard to health needs assessment. Their expertise and body of knowledge represents a unique resource in helping to achieve health gain, and the challenge they face is to ensure better understanding of how these skills address purchasers' and clients' needs.

Health visitors have unique skills and experience in delivering a range of services to help purchasers meet the objectives of *The Health of the Nation* (Department of Health, 1992) targets, the Children Act, the Patient's Charter and *Caring for People* (Department of Health, 1991a, 1991b, 1989 respectively). There is also evidence to suggest that where health visitors have been directly involved in discussions with purchasers, the service benefits have been more clearly understood (NHS Executive, 1994). However, it would appear that for the most effective use of health visitors to be achieved, health visitors and purchasers need to work together to adapt service priorities to changing national and local needs.

The key considerations to facilitate effective health promotion within the PHC setting involve a multifaceted approach, effective communication, teamworking, identification of priority groups and collaborative working. With the support and encouragement of FHSAs and a continuing high-profile debate to facilitate the sharing of experiences of good practice, the natural advantages of PHC can be complemented by realistic, relevant and sensitive approaches to health promotion. The banding arrangements for health promotion do not need to be seen as restrictive barriers, but can become flexible boundaries allowing both innovation and creativity.

References

Acheson, D. (1988). *Public Health in England*. London: HMSO.

Biddle, S., Fox, K. & Edmunds, L. (1994). *Physical Activity Promotion in Primary Health Care in England: Final Research Project for Health Education Authority*. London: Health Education Authority.

Black, D. & Townsend, P. (1982). *Inequalities in Health*. London: Penguin.

Brent Community Health Council (1981). *Black People and the Health Services*. Community Health Council, Brent.

Brown, P. (1995). GPs in poor areas 'losing 6m a year'. *The Guardian*, 4 January.

Calnan, M., Cant, S., Williams, S. & Killoran, A. (1994). Involvement of the primary health care team in coronary heart disease prevention. *British Journal of General Practice*, 44, 224–228.

Campbell, D. A., Radford, J. & Burton, P. (1991). Unemployment rates: an alternative to the Jarman index? *British Medical Journal* (28 September), *303*,750.

Carr-Hill, R., McIvor, S. & Dixon, P. (1989). *The NHS and its Customers.* Centre for Health Economics: University of York.

Cernik, K. and Wearne, M. (1991). Going public. *Primary health Care,* April.

Craft, N. & Dillner, L. (1994). GPs urgently need help in inner cities, says college. *British Medical Journal* (5 November), *309*.

Cupples, M. E. & McKnight, A. (1994). Randomised controlled trial of health promotion in general practice for patients at high cardiovascular risk. *British Medical Journal, 309*,993.

Daykin, N., Naidoo, J. & Wilson, N. (1995). *Effective Health Promotion in Primary Care.* Bristol: University of the West of England.

Department of Health (1989a). *General Practice in the National Health Service. The 1990 Contract.* London: HMSO.

Department of Health (1989b). *Caring for People: Community Care in the Next Decade and Beyond.* London : HMSO.

Department of Health (1991a). *Working Together Under the Children Act.* London: HMSO.

Department of Health (1991b). *The Patient's Charter.* London: HMSO.

Department of Health (1992). *The Health of the Nation: A Strategy for Health for England.* London: HMSO.

Department of Health (1993a). *Statement of Fees and Allowances Payable to GPs in England and Wales. London:* NHS Management Executive.

Department of Health (1993b). *Working Together for Better Health.* London: HMSO.

Department of Health (1993c). *On the State of the Public Health 1993.* London: HMSO.

Dowell, T. & Gosling, M. (1993). A practitioner perspective. In Health Education Authority, *Health Promotion and the Reforms in Primary* Health Care: A Review of HEA Policy, London: Health Education Authority.

Downie, R. S., Fyfe, C. & Tannahill, A. (1992). *Health Promotion Models and Values.* Oxford: Oxford University Press.

Ewles, L. (1996). The impact of the NHS reforms on specialist health promotion in the NHS. In A. Scriven & J. Orme (eds), *Health Promotion – Professional Perspectives.* London: Macmillan.

Family Heart Study Group (1994). Randomised controlled trial evaluating cardiovascular screening and intervention in general practice: principle results of the British Family Heart Study. *British Medical Journal* (29 January), *308*, 313–320.

French, J. (1990). Boundaries and horizons, the role of health education within health promotion. *Health Education Journal, 49*(1).

Garmston, A. (1994). Fit for 2000: cutting child accidents in Peacehavon. *Health Visitor, 67*(11).

General Services Medical Committee (1992). *The New Health Promotion Package.* London: British Medical Association.

Golding, P. (1986). *Excluding the Poor.* London: Child Poverty Action Group.

Hanlon, P., Toal, F. & Black, D. (1990). Health promotion under the new contract (letter). *British Journal of General Practice*, *40*, (349).

Health Education Authority (1991). *Primary Health Care Workshop Manual*. London: HEA.

Health Visitors' Association (1994). *Action for Health*. London: HVA.

Hunter, D. (1993). To market! To market!: a new dawn for community care? *Health and Social Care in the Community*, *1*(1).

Imperial Cancer Research Fund OXCHECK Study Group (1994). Effectiveness of health checks conducted by nurses in primary care: results of the OXCHECK study after one year. *British Medical Journal* (29 January), *308*, 308–312.

Ireland, R. (1996). Health promotion through leisure services. In A. Scriven & J. Orme (eds), *Health Promotion – Professional Perspectives*. London: Macmillan.

Jarman, B. (1983). Identification of underprivileged areas. *British Medical Journal*. *286*, 1706–1709.

Jelley, S. (1993). Prescription for health. *Healthlines*, April.

Kaufman, A. (1990). GPs crack under constant stress. *Physician*, *9*, 632–635.

Klein, R. (1992). *The Politics of the NHS*. London: Longman.

Labour Party (1989). *Meet the Challenge, Make the Change: Final Report of Labour Party Review for the 1990's*. London.

Main, J. & Main, P. (1990). Health checks in general practice (letter). *British Medical Journal*, 300, 1526.

Moores, Y. (1993). *New World, New Opportunities:Nursing in Primary Health Care*. London: National Health Service Management Executive.

Naidoo, J. & Wills, J. (1994). *Health Promotion Foundations for Practice*. London: Bailliere Tindall.

Naish, J. & Kline, R. (1990). What counts can't always be counted. *Health Visitor*, *13*(12).

NHS Executive (1994). *The Contribution of Health Visiting to Effective Purchasing*. Health Visitor Marketing Project Purchasers Report. London: NHSME.

Orme, J. (1994). *Health promotion in general practice – bands or boundaries*. Unpublished dissertation. Bristol: University of the West of England.

Orr, J. (1991). Making No Sense. *Health Visitor*, *64*(9).

Paris, J. A. G. & Player, D. (1993). Citizen's advice in general practice. *British Medical Journal*, (5 June) *306*, 1518–1520.

Pearson, M., Dawson, C., Moore, H. & Spence, S, (1993). Health on borrowed time?: Prioritising and meeting needs in low-income households. *Health and Social Care*, *1*(1).

Prentice, S. (1991). What will we find at the market? *Health Visitor*, *64*(1).

Royal College of General Practitioners (1991). *Report of the Inner City Task Force of the Royal College of General Practitioners*. Occasional Paper 66. London.

Stockport Health Authority (1993). Exercise on prescription. *Healthlines*, April.

Stott, N. (1993). When something is good, more of the same is not always better. *British Journal of General Practice*, *43*, 254–258.

Stott, N., Kinnersley, P. & Rollnick, S. (1994). The limits to health promotion. *British Medical Journal*, *309*, 971.

Tannahill, A. (1988). Editorial. *Community Medicine*, *10*, 94–97.

Tomlinson (1992). *Report of the Inquiry into London's Health Service, Medical Education and Research*. London: HMSO.

Tudor Hart, J. (1971). The inverse care law. *Lancet*, 1, *405–412*.

Watkins, S. (1991). Back to the roots. *Health Visitor*, *64*(10).

Williams, S., Calnan, M., Cant, L. & Coyle, J. (1993). All Change in the NHS?: Implications of the NHS reforms for primary care prevention. *Sociology of Health and Illness*, *15*(1).

World Health Organisation (1985). *Targets for Health for All*. Copenhagen: WHO.

World Health Organisation (1986). *Ottawa Charter for Health Promotion*. Geneva: WHO.

6 The impact of the NHS reforms on specialist health promotion in the NHS

Linda Ewles

It is possible to look back over decades of health promotion work in the NHS and see the long evolution of the specific NHS service we now call specialist health promotion (Ewles, 1993a). In earlier times, this service was more usually called a health education service, but as its remit expanded into areas of work not generally thought of as education, such as health policy development, it became known as health promotion and its professional staff changed their titles from health education or promotion officers to health promotion specialists.

The term specialist evolved to make the distinction between *generalist* and *specialist* health promotion services. Thinking about the generalist first, it is apparent that many people spend time in promoting health as part of their paid work, voluntary activity, or just as part of their day-to-day lives, such as parents bringing up their children in a healthy way of life (Ewles and Simnett, 1995). Those outside the health service include voluntary organisations, community and youth workers, teachers and environmental health officers. Those in the NHS include nurses, health visitors, doctors, dentists, dietitians, chiropodists and many other health care workers. At the forefront of preventive work in the NHS are those who work in community (as opposed to hospital) settings, with individuals, families and groups, aiming to make day-to-day living a healthier experience. All these people may be termed health promotion generalists because health promotion is an integral part, but not the whole, of what they do.

In contrast, health promotion specialists spend all their time in health promotion: planning, implementing and evaluating a range of health promotion activities. They are a body of skilled people with expertise in a wide range of health promotion work using varied approaches and methodologies.

The range of work covers the provision of expert support and training for generalist health promoters; supplying health education mate-

66

rials (such as information, public education leaflets, educational resources, display materials, teaching packs and audio-visual aids); running public awareness and education programmes; working with mass media; developing health promoting policies; and lobbying for healthy public policies. They provide a significant focus for coordinating, facilitating and often leading multi-agency (healthy alliance) work, crucial for successful implementation of national strategies for health such as *The Health of the Nation* (Department of Health, 1992). In many districts, they are the focus for preventive programmes in *Health of the Nation* priorities, known as Key Areas, and for broader-based programmes of community health development and work in settings such as schools and workplaces.

Health promotion specialists are usually based within community services or public health medicine departments (Society of Health Education and Health Promotion Specialists, 1993a). Their career pathways have generally started from a basis of professional training in health-related work, such as nursing or teaching, topped up with post-graduate qualifications and experience in health promotion.

It is important to recognise that the number of health promotion specialists is small compared with other disciplines within the NHS. The Society of Health Education and Health Promotion Specialists (SHEPS) estimates that there are around 1000 health promotion specialists in the UK (SHEPS, 1993b). Compare this with around 3600 registered dietitians or 25 000 registered physiotherapists, most of whom are considered to be in current practice (Council for Professions Supplementary to Medicine, 1994). Small departments of a few specialists and supporting staff have always been the norm, ever since the first health education departments were established in the 1950s. Departments where professional staff numbers run into double figures are only just becoming less of a rarity, but mainly because small departments are merging, not because of any dramatic overall increase in numbers.

To call specialist health promotion a profession is arguable, since specialised training is not a statutory obligation and there are no requirements for a license to practice as a prerequisite of employment, in the way that is required of, for example, nurses and dietitians. Whether to pursue the pathway to full professional status is a hotly debated issue within the health promotion specialists' professional body, SHEPS.

The points about small numbers and lack of statutory professional status are important when considering the impact of the NHS reforms on specialist health promotion. It is arguable that a larger body, with recognised professional status, would have fared better.

Changes as a result of the NHS reforms

The impact of the NHS reforms, set out in a White Paper in 1989 (Department of Health, 1989) and made statutory by the NHS and Community Care Act in 1990, sent waves of change reverberating through specialist health promotion services. These will be considered in three categories: organisational changes, new opportunities and constraints.

Organisational change: the purchaser/provider split

The changes which most affected specialist health promotion were concerned with organisational structure. Formerly, there was a District Health Promotion Officer who headed up a department of health promotion specialists. Crucially, the reforms brought the division between *purchasing* and *providing* functions. *Purchasers* (also known as *commissioners*) are the health authority bodies which assess health needs and purchase health services to meet those needs. They set contracts for services with *providers*. Providers are mainly community and hospital services now organised as self-governing NHS trusts.

Faced with this division, and the need to locate specialist health promotion services somewhere in the new structure, it was soon apparent that there was no obvious clear choice. On the one hand, health promotion specialists provided a service, therefore rightly belonging to the provider side of the fence. On the other hand, they did not provide a *direct patient* service, and they were strongly linked into public health medicine departments (seen from the first as purchasers). They had a role in needs assessment and strategic planning on a broad front, and worked extensively with agencies outside the NHS on developing health promotion strategies and programmes. Health promotion specialists initiated their own debates and discussed the pros and cons of a range of models (French and Adams, 1990), but there were no official guidelines or recommendations from, for example, the Department of Health or the Health Education Authority.

As a result, the issue was resolved locally in many different ways: some departments became providers in NHS Trusts or Directly Managed Units (DMUs) as part of community services; some became DMUs in their own right (sometimes called agencies), some remained with public health medicine as purchasers. Some split up, with one health promotion specialist, usually the former District Health Promotion Officer, becoming a purchaser and the rest becoming a provider service. Some evolved a dual role, undertaking both purchasing and providing functions (Linney, 1993).

The debate and the organisational changes are still going on in 1995, now informed by surveys and research studies (Society of Health Education and Promotion Specialists, 1993a; Smith 1993). There does not seem to be a clear pattern emerging and there is no published research evidence to indicate which model, if any, will prove to be the most effective in the long run.

These changes were profoundly unsettling, and continue to be so for many specialist health promotion services. Experience and observation suggests that the relationship of health promotion specialists across the purchaser–provider divide is varied: from the ideal of a relationship based on mutual respect, trust and collaboration, to one characterised by animosity, suspicion and power struggles.

Organisational change: the relationship with public health medicine

A key feature was the change in the relationship with public health medicine. For some, long-established links weakened for health promotion specialists who became providers when their public health medicine colleagues became purchasers. This meant a loss of expertise and support for health promotion programmes run by provider services. For others, an additional problem was the loss of the 'patronage' of public health medicine as health promotion specialists were left to fend for themselves in provider units, in competition for resources with other community and hospital services. Some found a new relationship with public health medicine was one of being controlled by contracts.

The move into NHS trusts was traumatic for some departments, which experienced a different style and management accountability.

Organisational change: mergers

Another common structural change was that some health education/ promotion departments became subject to mergers, either because their parent health authorities merged into larger purchasing health authorities or health commissions, or because purchasing health authorities sought to rationalise and strengthen the small departments they had inherited on their 'patch'. Mergers upset established allegiances, networks and ways of working, both inside and outside the NHS.

The impact of these organisational changes, often taking years to agree and settle, should not be underestimated. Such issues sap energy and channel resources into sheer survival, rather than into the development of services for the benefit of the population. Furthermore, the key agencies with whom health promotion specialists work, notably local authorities, were undergoing their own organisational changes at the same time, compounding the difficulties.

Opportunities: the contract culture

However, the NHS reforms also brought opportunities which some health promotion specialists picked up with enthusiasm. Health promotion could be written into contracts as a requirement, rather than being a low-status optional extra (Killoran, 1992). The impression is that by 1995 most health authorities require health promotion as part of their provider service contracts. Guidelines have been produced, often on specific subjects (Alcohol Concern, 1991; Health Education Authority, 1994).

Specifications for health promotion are often written into contracts in three ways. First, there can be a general requirement that NHS services promote the health of staff and patients by providing, for example, smoke-free environments, healthy food, and good-quality patient information. Second, there can be a health promotion requirement linked to specific services, such as a requirement that maternity services should provide advice and help for pregnant women to stop smoking. Third, specialist health promotion services can be contracted to provide a range of services, such as training, resource services, and specific programmes on topics such as HIV prevention or work in settings such as schools.

The need for a contract for a specialist health promotion service has meant hard thinking about exactly what that service should provide. Of necessity, thinking has also sharpened up on quality standards in health promotion, value for money and cost effectiveness (Society of Health Education and Promotion Specialists, 1992; Tolley, 1994). There is increasing pressure to define clearly what health promotion activity *achieves*. From the commissioner's point of view, the question raised is (crudely), 'what health improvement in our population are we getting in return for our investment in specialist health promotion services?' It was, and still is, a time for re-evaluating the service traditionally provided, and introducing changes. New research has been instigated into defining quality standards and evaluating effectiveness (Evans *et al.*, 1994; Speller and Funnell, 1994).

Effort has also been channelled into developing methods for monitoring a contract for health promotion services, to be used by the new breed of commissioners. A health service culture of looking for *quantitative* measures has developed, such as morbidity rates, numbers of operations and finished consultant episodes (FCEs), but health promotion does not sit easily with this approach. There is no neat unit of measurement, parallel to an FCE, which can be applied right across the range of activities. This means that there is no clear way of monitoring *how much* health promotion activity is underway. This is also recognised as difficult in other services too, such as community health work, but the search goes on in, for example, measuring activity in health visiting and district nurse work. There is a trend to specify quantified targets in programmes of work, no doubt initiated by the emphasis on targets in *The Health of the Nation*.

For some, an issue has emerged about how health promotion specialists present health promotion to others, such as commissioners, managers and board members (professional and lay) on health authorities and NHS Trusts. Traditionally, the emphasis has been on describing activity, perhaps with an underlying assumption that people will unquestioningly accept that such activity is a good thing. Often they do not – health promotion can be seen as unwelcome 'nannying', coming from do-gooding spoilsports with negative messages, wasting public money because people don't respond anyway, and curbing freedom of the individual. This has pointed up a need to learn how to present health promotion in terms of outcomes rather than activities, with much clearer rationale. Commissioners want to know what has been achieved with their investment; in other words, the outcomes rather than the details of processes.

So the contract culture has brought opportunities to specify health promotion in contracts, and this provided the impetus to sharpen up on defining outcomes, targets and quality standards; identifying evidence of effectiveness and value for money; and developing monitoring methods and units of activity measurement.

It is worth mentioning that the coincidental advent of national strategies for health in the early 1990s also drove these changes forward: *The Health of the Nation* in England, and comparable strategies in Scotland, Wales and Northern Ireland (Department of Health, 1992). These strategies were significant, as it was the first time a strategy for *health*, as opposed to health *services*, had ever been produced. This gave health promotion a higher profile, and put added pressure on health commissioners to ensure that health promotion strategies were devised and programmes commissioned to meet *The Health of the Nation* targets. It also put pressure on health promotion specialist providers to deliver those programmes.

Opportunities: resource shifts

The theory that purchasing health authorities could commission more health promotion services if they so wished, and commit themselves to prevention in the teeth of the traditional heavy lobby for treatment and cure services, meant that there was a theoretical opportunity to shift resources from treatment to prevention. This ability to shift resources has proved difficult in practice, and it is hard to identify much extra investment in health promotion since the NHS reforms. This is not surprising as pressures to keep costs down are tremendous, and there was no new money to support *The Health of the Nation*.

Constraints: competitive ethos

The NHS reforms are underpinned by a belief that market forces and competition will lead to more efficient, effective health services. But this poses a fundamental problem for specialist health promotion work (Ewles, 1993b). Health promotion practice is deeply rooted in an ethos of collaboration, which is specifically encouraged in *Health of the Nation* and other documents (Department of Health, 1993). The strains imposed by competition and conflicts of interest are often very uncomfortable indeed. Promoting health for a defined population, such as a city or a county, will involve purchaser health authorities (possibly more than one) and a range of providers from NHS Trusts. Some of these are likely to be in competition with one another for health authority funds, and colleagues who have worked together for many years on health promotion projects may now find themselves competing for contracts (Evans and Ewles, 1994).

Furthermore, most alliance work does not split neatly into purchasing and providing; multi-agency groups usually straddle the whole range of needs assessment, goal-setting, planning, implementing and evaluating health promotion programmes. There is no tidy divide into purchasing and providing, so both need to sit round the table. This adds to the confusion of other agencies, who (like most of the population) are only just beginning to comprehend the complexities of commissioning, Trusts, contracts, fundholding and the rest. Furthermore, an alliance where two or more of the parties are already in a contractual arrangement is an uncomfortable added dynamic in multi-agency working.

Looking to the future

To summarise, the NHS reforms brought changes, opportunities and constraints for specialist health promotion services. There were significant organisational changes, which disrupted services and absorbed energy for many years. There were opportunities to develop health promotion as a feature of the new health service contracts, but strains were imposed by the necessity to work within an infrastructure designed for competition rather than collaboration.

Other changes loom which raise important questions. For example, what will be the impact, if any, of the trend to tighten contracting and monitoring further, as has happened in acute services, where *floors* and *ceilings* for volumes of work are tightly defined (NHS Executive, 1994a)? What will happen as a result of increased GP fundholding (NHS Executive, 1994b)? If it increases to the point that health commissions have little left to commission themselves, will they 'topslice' for specialist health promotion, or will the funding become dependent on the views of GPs? Will local authorities take on specialist health promotion work, leaving the NHS to deal solely with treatment and care?

In the face of so many unknowns, it is only possible to speculate on the future of specialist health promotion services in the NHS. But it is arguable that their future depends on the key ingredients of increased professionalism, evidence of effectiveness, investment in larger departments and a prolonged period of organisational stability.

References

Alcohol Concern (1991). *Contracting for Alcohol Services*. London: Alcohol Concern.

Council for Professions Supplementary to Medicine (1994). *Annual Report*. London: CPSM.

Department of Health (1989). *Working for Patients*. London: HMSO.

Department of Health (1992). *The Health of the Nation*. London: HMSO.

Department of Health (1993). *Working Together for Better Health*. London: HMSO.

Evans, D. & Ewles, L. (1994). A leap in the dark. *Health Service Journal, 104* (5410), 30–31.

Evans, D., Head, M. & Speller, V. (1994). *Assuring Quality in Health Promotion – How to Develop Standards of Good Practice*. London: Wessex Institute of Public Health Medicine in collaboration with the Health Education Authority.

Ewles, L. (1993a). Paddling upstream for 50 years: the role of health education officers. *Health Education Journal, 53*(3), 172–181.

Ewles, L. (1993b). Hope Against Hype. *Health Service Journal, 103*(5367), 30–31.

Ewles, L. & Simnett, I. (1995). *Promoting Health – A Practical Guide*, 3rd ed. London: Scutari Press. Chapter 4.

French, J. & Adams, L. (1990). *Health Promotion in the 90s: Organisational Options for Health Promotion Services*. Workshop Report. London: King's Fund Institute.

Health Education Authority (1994). *Contracts for Smoking Prevention – Current Practice in the NHS*. London: Health Education Authority.

Killoran, A. (1992). *Putting Health into Contracts*. London: Health Education Authority.

Linney, J. (1993). Gain without pain. *The Health Service Journal*, *103*(5349), 29–30.

NHS Executive (1994a). *1995-96 Contracting Review Handbook*, Leeds: Department of Health.

NHS Executive (1994b). *1995-96 Developing NHS Purchasing and GP Fundholding – Towards a Primary Care-led NHS*. Leeds: Department of Health.

Smith, D. (1993). *Options for the Future: Organisational Arrangements for Health Promotion Services*. London: Health Education Authority.

Society of Health Education and Health Promotion Specialists (1992). *Developing Quality in Health Education and Health Promotion -- A Manual for all Those Involved in the Delivery of a Quality Service*. Sheffield: SHEPS.

Society of Health Education and Health Promotion Specialists (1993a). *Health Promotion at the Crossroads: A Study of Health Promotion Departments in the Reorganised NHS*. Sheffield: SHEPS.

Society of Health Education and Health Promotion Specialists (1993b). Personal communication.

Speller, V. & Funnell, R. (1994). *Towards Evaluating Health Alliances. HEA Multi-Sectoral Collaboration for Health: Evaluation Project. Phase 1*. London: Health Education Authority and Wessex Institute of Public Health Medicine.

Tolley, K. (1994). *Health Promotion: How to Measure Cost-effectiveness*. London: Health Education Authority.

7 The potential for health promotion in hospital nursing practice

Sue Latter

In recent decades there has been a rise in consumerism in matters pertaining to health, as well as changes in patterns of disease and a shift towards self-care and management of illness and rehabilitation in the community. This has been combined with an increased emphasis on a holistic model of health within nursing, incorporating psychological and social as well as physical dimensions. The result has been a recognition that nursing needs to move beyond its traditional function of caring for the sick and embrace an expanded role in health promotion. This is reflected in a number of recent strategic and policy documents (United Kingdom Central Council, 1986; Royal College of Nursing, 1989; Department of Health, 1989).

Whilst the health promotion function of nurses working in primary health care settings enjoys a longer tradition, it is only latterly that this has been applied to nurses working in hospitals. The potential contribution of hospital nurses to health promotion has been ill defined, as evidenced by the dearth of literature and empirical work available in this area. Many of the concepts central to health promotion are more readily applicable to the community or primary care setting than to the hospital context. For example, the application of key health promotion activities in the hospital context such as building healthy public policy, creating supportive environments and strengthening community action (WHO, 1986) is a challenging task. In addition, values central to health promotion – collaboration, public participation and empowerment – do not sit easily with the tradition of hospital health care. The latter has been founded on a medical model approach to care, characterised by an orientation towards cure, on treatment in the medical environment, a tendency to dismiss the patient's perspective and an expectation of the patient's role as one which involves passivity, trust and a willingness to wait for medical help (Hart, 1991). However, these difficulties must be overcome and new ways of working, across traditional boundaries, will need to occur if hospital nurses are to be responsive to current and future

75

health care needs of the communities of people with whom they work. The vast number of hospital nurses, and their close and continuous contact with patients during an episode of heightened awareness about their health and illness, suggests that they have a powerful potential contribution to make to the health promotion movement.

An exploration of opportunities available for health promotion in hospital nursing practice follows below. The role of nurses as health educators with patients is first reviewed. This is followed by an analysis of the potential contribution of nurses to collaborative work on health issues at a broader, health promotion level. Constraints which may militate against achievement of this potential are also highlighted.

Hospital nurses as health educators

Currently, the focus of hospital nurses' work often revolves around care for the individual patient. Therefore, an important element of their health promotion potential concerns the health education interactions that they may engage in with patients. Some models of health promotion (for example, Tannahill, 1985; Tones, 1987) make clear that health education is a vital component of a broader health promotion strategy. There is now some consensus in the health promotion literature that individual education comprises an element of health promotion, together with action at a broader structural or policy level (Macdonald and Bunton, 1992). Historically, this aspect of the hospital nurse's role in health promotion has been enacted in the form of patient education about disease management and structured information given to patients in preparation for a stressful procedure. There exists a substantial body of empirical evidence to suggest that these activities have beneficial health outcomes, in the form of, for example, reduced anxiety and improved recovery rates. However, they represent only a limited aspect of the potential role of nurses in health education, in that they focus on illness management as opposed to health *per se*. Additionally, these activities have tended to be characterised by an emphasis on compliance (Wilson-Barnett and Osborne, 1983; Redman, 1993) and by didactic, standardised approaches (Wilson-Barnett, 1988). More recently, the need to adopt more individualised, patient-centred approaches, incorporating a recognition of the importance of self-efficacy beliefs and the wider barriers to taking health action has been noted (Wilson-Barnett, 1988; Secker-Walker, 1990; Vaughan, 1991; Redman, 1993). A focus on health-related interactions and the need to empower rather than coerce patients to comply would also seem in keeping with current health promotion philosophy and concepts.

Further aspects of the role of hospital nurses in health education can be outlined by drawing on current theoretical literature. For example,

Tones' (1987) model of health promotion depicts an educational component referred to as 'critical consciousness raising'. This refers to the idea that through a health education encounter, individuals may be encouraged to think critically about their lives and circumstances, and the health educator may raise awareness of the wider factors which determine health choices. This may then lead to collective action at a community level which pressurises those with power to adopt more health promoting policies. Draper's (1983) analysis of types of health education information also indicates further areas that hospital nurses need to consider as part of their health education role. He outlines the provision of information about preventive health services, education about the environment and how this influences health, and education about the politics of health as legitimate forms of health education. It is possible to suggest that there may be opportunities for hospital nurses to engage in dialogues of this nature with patients as part of their health promotion potential. A final strand to this health education role is highlighted by Downie *et al.*'s (1991) contention that health education involves not only communication activity with members of the community or general public (in this case patients), but it is also aimed at professionals and those with power. Maglacas (1988) also argues that nurses have a role in this, and suggests that nurses need to understand the agendas and priorities of key decision makers and to communicate effectively with them in the interests of having an impact on policies which influence health. An example in the hospital context might be that a nurse working on a care-for-the-elderly ward liaises with the local authority social services department over the need to allocate increased resources to home adaptations in order to prevent falls among the elderly.

Research which enables definitive statements to be made about the extent to which nurses in hospitals enact elements of this health education role is scarce. However, recent work by Macleod Clark *et al.* (1992) suggests that the reality falls short of the potential. Observation of nursing practice on six wards employed as case studies revealed varying degrees of integration of health education into nurses' work. Overall, however, there was a tendency for education to be disease orientated and standardised, with a lack of evidence that nurses were engaging patients in dialogue about wider health issues or communicating with other professionals and policy makers about health promotion issues.

Expanding the health promotion role for hospital nurses

Current health promotion policies and health service changes necessitate a reconsideration of traditional patterns of hospital nursing work.

That is, nurses' potential contribution to health promotion includes involvement in activities over and above their bedside health education interactions with patients. Whilst these will remain an important element of their role, there is a need to embrace new ways of working which are consistent with health promotion concepts and principles. Nurses need to recognise and develop their potential role in the broader arena of health promotion, in addition to their more traditional role as health educators. Creating environments which are supportive of health, encouraging community participation in health matters and helping to build healthy policies may all form part of the potential for health promotion in hospital nursing practice. However, this will not be achieved by nurses alone and highlights the need to work in partnership with others across traditional boundaries. The WHO (1985) makes clear that multisectoral cooperation is required for health promotion and calls on the health sector to open channels between itself and broader social, political, economic and physical environmental components. Recent UK health service legislation and policy may create opportunities for collaborative working. The UK Government has outlined its importance by recommending the need for healthy alliances, joint action and better coordination of the range of departments and agencies in pursuit of the targets outlined in *The Health of the Nation* White Paper (1992). It has also been suggested that the NHS Community Care Act (1991) represents a mechanism for achieving collaboration with other key agencies via its inception of purchaser and provider roles. Naidoo and Wills (1994) propose that part of the contracts and service specifications produced by purchasing DHAs may include certain standards of health education and promotion such as a smoke-free environment or the provision of healthy catering for NHS employees. The implication is that these standards will require collaboration between the various agencies involved, including nurses. The formation of alliances with other sectors, other professionals or voluntary groups requires a vision by hospital nurses of ways of working beyond the traditional boundaries of the bedside and of the ward itself.

Before considering the opportunities available for developing this aspect of hospital nursing practice, it is necessary to be clear about the contribution that this group of professionals can make to collaborative work for health. Whilst it is evident that responsibility for health promotion does not rest with the health sector alone, nurses nevertheless have a unique contribution to make to alliances created in pursuit of promoting health. Their close and continuous contact with patients and their carers inevitably gives a detailed and holistic understanding of their physical, psychological and social needs and the extent to which these are met by current service provision. For example, a nurse working on a gynaecological ward might identify a need for psychological support from others in the form of a miscarriage support group. Hospital nurses are also in a position to identify particular patterns and trends in admissions and can thus contribute their perspective to an assessment of local health needs. Nurses' specialised knowledge of health, the management of disease processes and prevention of complications also means that they are well placed to contribute to education and awareness-raising exercises within the hospital or broader community.

Collaborative working within the hospital

Opportunities for collaborative working for health exist within the hospital environment and also extend beyond its boundaries to the local community in which it is situated. Within the hospital, there is a need for nurses to engage with others in the process of creating and implementing policies which promote health. Examples of relevant policies include those set up to ensure smoke-free zones or those that promote healthy food choices for both patients and staff. Milz and Vang (1989) also comment on the contribution that architectural planning can make to a health promoting hospital by considering patients' needs for rest, calm, social communication and recreational activities. They also suggest that hospital surroundings should be ecologically safe and stimulating, and that patient and employer participation in the functioning of the system is an important component of health promotion. These exemplify areas in which nurses can bring their perspective to bear in pursuit of policies which promote health within the hospital.

The establishment of patient or carer groups represents a further mechanism for promoting health in hospitals, and may also provide opportunities for nurses to collaborate with other agencies or disciplines. In mapping out the repertoire of health promotion, Beattie (1991) suggests that a *personal counselling for health* approach may involve help provided through processes occurring within a group of peers with a group leader. Such groups may have a supportive and/or an educative function and nurses may have a role as initiators, facilitators or occasional contributors, depending on the nature of the group itself. With the trend towards shorter admission periods for patients, it becomes increasingly necessary to consider new ways of meeting patients' and carers' needs. The establishment of groups for patients or carers with similar needs, either in the pre-admission or the post-discharge period, represents one way forward. They may also present an opportunity for collaboration with others engaged in health promotion work. A good example is the recent proliferation of cardiac rehabilitation groups for patients who have experienced a myocardial infarction or cardiac surgery. The nature of these vary widely, but they are often characterised by multi-disciplinary educational input from specialists such as dieticians, physiotherapists and counsellors, as well as nurses. Nurses' insight into the experiences patients are likely to encounter during their admission and their knowledge of the requirements of the rehabilitation process means that they can make a valuable contribution to such groups.

Collaboration with the community

The potential for health promotion in hospital nursing practice also includes liaison and collaboration with agencies working to promote health in the community. Recent trends in health care have contributed to a breaking down of the boundaries which once established hospitals as discrete institutions isolated from the broader community. The NHS Community Care Act (Department of Health, 1991a) means hospital personnel need to be cognisant of local health care needs upon which contracts with purchasing authorities are based. Increasingly rapid turnover of patients, together with the commitment that the hospital will agree arrangements for meeting patients' discharge needs with agencies such as community nursing services and local authority social services departments (Department of Health, 1991b), creates a need for greater collaboration. Robinson (1994) also comments on the changing boundaries of the American hospital. He suggests that accountable health partnerships that emphasise outpatient, home health and sub-acute care could, 'provide a window of opportunity for the hospital to embark on a new mission as a health care center without walls'. All this points to a need to reconsider traditional boundaries of hospital nursing work and to create partnerships with other agencies in pursuit of health promotion.

The hospital is a part of the community in which it is situated, and health promotion initiatives should be based on this principle. Milz and Vang (1989) suggest that a new, positive vision for hospitals in the promotion of health incorporates broadening and strengthening communication with the community at large. They highlight the need to integrate the hospital's special concerns into the wider health promotion efforts of various institutions and levels of government in the community. One way in which this might be achieved is through the hospital playing a role in local coalitions and strategies as part of the WHO Healthy Cities initiative. Hospital-wide health promotion initiatives also present opportunities for the formation of alliances. These are recommended by McBride and Moorwood (1994) as more effective than those involving isolated wards, as they have the potential to be more cost-effective, encourage multi-disciplinary participation and allow cross-fertilization of ideas between staff from different patient areas. They may also allow collaborative working with agencies in the community. For example, a focus on the hospital as a health-promoting environment might involve nurses liaising with other disciplines within the hospital such as occupational health and catering managers as well as local authority environmental health officers and planners, the local media and lay members of the community.

Alternatively, another way in which hospital nurses might work collaboratively is by going out into the community and sharing their knowledge and expertise. An example of this came to light in a recent research study (Macleod Clark *et al.*, 1992). A ward sister working on a specialist ward for neuro-muscular disorders liaised regularly with the local support group for those affected by multiple sclerosis and gave talks to interested members on aspects of disease management. She also spoke to local womens' and church groups on various topics associated with neuro-muscular disorders. Additionally, collaboration existed such that volunteer workers from local support groups visited patients and carers on the ward who were in need of support.

Available empirical data suggests that nurses' involvement in collaborative work for health is limited. With the exception of the example cited above, Macleod Clark *et al.*'s (1992) study of health promotion in hospital nursing practice revealed scant evidence of collaborative working, away from direct care-giving at the bedside. From an interview sample of 132 ward sisters, only one or two isolated examples emerged: one ward sister reported formal liaison with a local Health Promotion Officer and the hospital catering manager with a view to influencing the menu choices available in the hospital. Another had been asked to join a multi-disciplinary District Health Authority working party on nutrition policy. Whilst not focusing exclusively on hospital nurses, a study by Gott and O'Brien (1990a) revealed a similar picture. Their findings illustrated a nursing approach to health promotion orientated around the provision of individualistic lifestyle advice and a lack of shared policies or broader action strategies for health promotion.

The way forward

If hospital nursing practice is to move forward towards the potential outlined here, a number of issues will need to be addressed. As a starting point, nurses require a sound understanding of the meaning of the concepts of health education and health promotion and their application to the hospital setting. Progress towards fulfilling this potential also dictates that nurses are equipped with relevant skills which enable them to take action. At the level of health education with individual patients, there must be a recognition of central concepts such as empowerment and holism, as well as the need for individualised approaches. Appropriate interpersonal skills are needed to operationalise these concepts in practice. Working with others to promote health beyond the bedside also requires an informed understanding of health promotion concepts and principles. As Cribb and Dines (1993) point out, when individuals are operating with different and conflicting personal models of health promotion, this can act as a barrier to effective communication. The Health of the Nation handbook (Department of Health, 1993) on healthy alliances also identifies the need for a shared vision and concept of health as an important first step. Nurses will also need to be proficient in skills such as those outlined by Naidoo and Wills (1994) including communication, participation in meetings, managing paperwork and time and being and working in a group.

Recent research (Latter, 1994) highlighted that hospital nurses were operating with very limited perceptions of health education and health promotion which were akin to illness-oriented, individualistic approaches. Findings indicated that there was generally a lack of recognition of the broader policy or structural aspect of health promotion, and none of those interviewed made reference to the principle of intersectoral collaboration as part of their understanding of health promotion. Nevertheless, opportunities are emerging to address this deficit in understanding. Within nurse education, a central aim of the pre-registration Project 2000 (UK Central Council for Nurses, 1986) curriculum is to equip nurses of the future for their role as health promoters, based on a sound understanding of health promotion theory. Qualified, practising nurses are also able to update their knowledge and skills in health promotion through, for example, accessing relevant courses offered as part of the English National Board for Nursing, Midwifery and Health Visiting's (1991) Higher Award Framework.

However, education about health promotion knowledge and skills is unlikely, by itself, to be sufficient to enable nurses to fulfil their potential in hospital settings. Enacting the strategies outlined above will also necessitate a consideration of new ways of working over and above the historical focus on ward specialities and care delivered to individual patients. Grasping opportunities for collaboration and the forging of healthy alliances means working across ward and hospital boundaries which have been created as a consequence of a focus on illness as opposed to health promotion. The Department of Health (1993) identifies the need for support for collaborative working and the necessity of a mechanism for making progress. As well as informal networking, in the hospital setting organisational structures need to be established and supported whereby multi-agency work on health promotion issues is possible. This might involve nurse management representation on multi-disciplinary or multi-agency health promotion committees or forums.

A final issue which will need to be addressed concerns the status and autonomy of nurses. If nurses are to empower patients as part of their health education role, and work in collaboration with other key players in the promotion of health, then it is essential that they are invested with the authority and autonomy to do so. Pearson (1988) suggests that autonomy for patients means autonomy for nurses because otherwise the nurse who is with the patient is powerless to allow them to carry out the decisions they make. Tones (1993) also makes this connection clear. He states that any policy designed to achieve a health promoting hospital should not overlook the fact that a hospital comprises a community of both patients *and* staff. Therefore, its aim should be to empower not only patients, but staff too. Status and authority to influence organisational decisions are also a prerequisite for successful collaborative ventures with other groups or agencies involved in health promotion. Historically, nurses have not enjoyed such status or authority, either individually or collectively. As Gott and O'Brien (1990b) highlight, the nursing profession has near universal subordinate status *vis-à-vis* other professions and interests, and nurses are afforded little authority or control in a health care system dominated by the priorities of its superordinate allied professions. Tones' (1993) suggestion that assertiveness training should form part of the nurse education curriculum to support their health promotion function and contribute to their sense of professional identity is relevant here. Perhaps what is also required are systems of nurse education which foster empowerment, and a philosophy of practice which values the centrality of nursing expertise, as well as systems of care organisation which allow individual nurses the power to make decisions and act on these.

To conclude, as nursing moves towards the 21st century, it must re-evaluate traditional methods of delivering health care and create new ways of working which are congruent with current health trends and policy changes. The potential for health promotion in hospital nursing practice includes both health education with individual patients and working across professional boundaries to collaborate with others in the spirit of health promotion. Nurses need education in health promotion knowledge and skills, as well as organisational structures within the hospital to enable collaborative working on health issues. Increased status and autonomy for the nursing profession is also needed in order that nurses can fulfil their health promotion potential.

References

Beattie, A. (1991). Knowledge and control in health promotion: a test case for social policy and social theory. In J. Gabe, M. Calnan & M. Bury (eds), *The Sociology of the Health Service*. London: Routledge.

Cribb, A. & Dines, A. (1993). What is health promotion? In A. Dines & A. Cribb (eds), *Health Promotion: Concepts and Practice*. Oxford: Blackwell Scientific.

Department of Health (1989). *A Strategy for Nursing*. Department of Health Nursing Division. London: HMSO.

Department of Health (1991a). *The NHS and the Community Care Act*. London: HMSO.

Department of Health (1991b). *The Patients' Charter*. London: HMSO.

Department of Health (1992). *The Health of the Nation*. London: HMSO.

Department of Health (1993). *The Working Together for Better Health*. London: HMSO.

Downie, R. S., Fyfe, C. & Tannahill, A. (1991). *Health Promotion: Models and Values*. (Revised reprint). Oxford: Oxford Medical Publications.

Draper, P. (1983). Tackling the disease of ignorance. *Self-Health*, 1, 23–25.

English National Board for Nursing (1991). *The Higher Award Framework*. London: English National Board for Nursing.

Gott, M. & O'Brien, M. (1990a). Practice and the prospect for change. *Nursing Standard*, 10(5), 30–32.

Gott, M. & O'Brien, M. (1990b). *The Role of the Nurse in Health Promotion: Policies, Perspectives and Practice*. Report of a two-year research project funded by the Department of Health, Department of Health and Social Welfare. Milton Keynes: Open University.

Hart, N. (1991). *The Sociology of Health and Medicine*. Ormskirk, Lancashire: Causeway Press.

Latter, S. (1994). Health education and health promotion: perceptions and practice of nurses in acute care settings. Unpublished PhD thesis, King's College, University of London.

Macleod Clark, J., Wilson-Barnett, J., Latter, S. & Maben, J. (1992). *Health Education and Health Promotion in Nursing: A Study of Practice in Acute Areas*. Report of a two-year research project funded by the Department of Health, Department of Nursing Studies. King's College: University of London.

Macdonald, G. & Bunton, R. (1992). Health promotion: discipline or disciplines? In R. Bunton & G. Macdonald (eds), *Health Promotion: Disciplines and Diversity*. London: Routledge.

Maglacas, A. M. (1988). Health for all: nursing's role. *Nursing Outlook*, 36(2), 66–71.

McBride, A. & Moorwood, Z. (1994). The hospital health promotion facilitator: an evaluation. *Journal of Clinical Nursing*, 3, 355–359.

Milz, H. & Vang, J. O. (1989). Consultation on the role of health promotion in hospitals. *Health Promotion*, 3(4), 425–427.

Naidoo, J. & Wills, J. (1994). *Health Promotion: Foundations for Practice*. London: Balliere Tindall.

Pearson, A. (ed) (1988). *Primary Nursing: Nursing in the Burford and Oxford Nursing Development Units*. London: Croom Helm.

Redman, B. K. (1993). Patient education at 25 Years: where we have been and where we are going. *Journal of Advanced Nursing*, 18 (5), 725–730.

Robinson, J. C. (1994). The changing boundaries of the American hospital. *The Milbank Quarterly, 72*(2), 259–275.

Royal College of Nursing (1989). *Into The Nineties: Promoting Professional Excellence*. London: Royal College of Nursing.

Secker-Walker, R. H. (1990). Commentary. In S. Schumaker, E. B. Schron & J. K. Ockene (eds), *The Handbook of Health Behaviour Change*. New York: Springer.

Tannahill, A. (1985). What is health promotion? *Health Education Journal, 44*, 167–168.

Tones, K. (1987). Promoting health: the contribution of education. Paper presented at the World Health Organization Consultation on the Co-ordinated Infrastructure for Health Education, Copenhagen.

Tones, K. (1993). The theory of health promotion: implications for nursing. In J. Wilson-Barnett & J. Macleod Clark (eds), *Research in Health Promotion and Nursing*. London: Macmillan.

United Kingdom Central Council for Nurses, Midwives and Health Visitors (1986). *Project 2000*. London: UKCC.

Vaughan, B. (1991). Patient education in therapeutic nursing. In R. McMahon & A. Pearson (eds), *Nursing as Therapy*, 1st ed. London: Chapman and Hall.

Wilson-Barnett, J. (1988). Patient teaching or patient counselling? *Journal of Advanced Nursing, 13*(2), 215–222.

Wilson-Barnett, J. & Osborne, J. (1983). Studies evaluating patient teaching: implications for practice. *International Journal of Nursing Studies, 20*(1), 33–43.

World Health Organization (1985). *Targets for Health for All*. Copenhagen: WHO Regional Office for Europe.

World Health Organization (1986). *Ottawa Charter for Health Promotion*. Ottawa, Canada: WHO.

SECTION THREE

Local authority

8 Health promotion, environmental health and the local authority

Peter Allen

The Health of the Nation (Department of Health, 1992) recognises that local authorities are responsible for a wide range of public services, many of which are linked with the strategy set out in the white paper. These responsibilities include education, environmental control, environmental health and food safety, transport, housing and social services. This chapter looks at what local authorities can do to advance health in particular through their environmental health officers (EHOs).

The difference between local government authorities and health authorities

There is a significant difference between local government authorities and health authorities. In the health authorities, accountability is predominantly upwards to the Secretary of State with her\his enormous powers to make key appointments and make available financial resources. On the other hand accountability in local government is predominantly downward to local people. Healthy alliances between the two types of authorities are crucial if health is to be effectively promoted. If a health authority tries to work in isolation with regard to health promotion, without linking with the local authority it foregoes the unique relationship that exists between the town hall and its local people. Furthermore, if a local authority distances itself from the health authority, it misses out on the wider perspective, particularly the expertise and relevant experience.

Another important point that needs to be made is that local authorities like health authorities have dynamic structures which are subject to frequent change. The present situation in local government is that although in some larger urban areas, such as Birmingham and London, local government is arranged on a single-tier principle, in most other places local government is divided up into two tiers. This has an important implication for health promotion because it can mean that important health promotion services such as education and social services (which will be examined in later chapters) are in one local authority – a county council – and other equally important health promotion services such as housing and environmental health are in another – a district council. This can lead to duplication, confusion, misunderstandings and waste of resources.

In an attempt to overcome this two-tier approach, the Local Government Commission was set up in 1991 with the aim of introducing single-tier or *unitary* authorities. However, its initial findings make it clear that the two-tier system of local government will continue for at least the foreseeable future and so local government health promotion services will continue to be provided on a split basis. This should not discourage health promotion practitioners. It is simply making clear that we need to take the concept of healthy alliances to a deeper level and see the need for its application not just between local authorities, health authorities and others, but between local authorities and between the different professionals that make up local government.

Role models

Before examining environmental health services which are the main focus of this chapter, it is worth making one further point. In England and Wales there are over 400 local authorities with nearly two and a half million employees. In terms of the employment market this is a substantial segment. If local authorities take action to introduce effective health policies they can not only provide their internal community with an opportunity for better health, but they can also provide a role model for local commerce and industry. Many have followed this approach on specific health promotion issues.

The Institution of Environmental Health Officers (IEHO), carried out a survey to establish the situation as regards smoking. They found that 85 per cent of local authorities that responded had in fact established non-smoking policies. To help local authorities, the IEHO with the Health Education Authority (HEA) have published guidelines for smoking policies in local authorities (Institute of Environmental Health Officers, 1993). Their booklet contains a step-by-step guide as well as much other useful information. Local authorities can therefore act as local role models in a wide range of health aspects from balanced alcohol policies to good green practice.

The contribution of local authority environmental health services to health promotion

There was a time when it was argued that health promotion and enforcement were different entities. Today, that argument sounds a bit hollow. Increasingly health promotion is seen as an umbrella term to cover all interventions that promote health including enforcement. As Tones (1990) puts it, health promotion incorporates all measures deliberately designed to promote health and handle disease.

The environmental health enforcement duties of local authorities are set out in legislation, and cover:

- Food inspection and food hygiene and safety;
- Housing standards;
- Health and safety at work and during recreation;
- Environmental protection including statutory nuisances;
- Communicable disease prevention and control;
- Licensing;
- Drinking water surveillance;
- Refuse collection and street cleansing;
- Pest control.

A detailed description of these duties is set out in the environmental health officers handbook (Bassett, 1991). However, as far as health promotion is concerned, what needs to be noted is that the above mandatory enforcement duties are vital if health is to be advanced. For example, people need sound and adequate housing. It is inappropriate to simply provide a first-class primary health care service and new hospitals if adequate and suitable housing is not provided. Nor does it make sense in economic terms. Illness caused by poor housing is estimated to cost the NHS £2 billion a year (Standing Conference on Public Health, 1994). This has obvious implications for our limited national health service resources.

Discretionary powers

Environmental health officers also have an extensive range of discretionary powers. See, for instance, those detailed in section 54 of the Public Health Act 1964 and the Home Safety Act of 1961. These discretionary powers can make a significant contribution to health promotion. In recent years, work carried out under these sections cover such topics as HIV\AIDS, alcohol and drug addiction, nutrition, women's health, men's health, heating and energy advice, occupational health, health aspects of poverty, greening, health grants to voluntary organisations and of course the range of varied activities covered by home safety.

An example of how a local authority through its discretionary powers can promote health can be seen in the Oxford Airwatch Partnership Project. In the early 1990s, the Oxford City Council was faced with growing concern about ill health caused by traffic. It was also faced like other local authorities with ambivalent standards. Firstly there was pollution. No money to monitor the effects: the Government had funded a handful of monitoring stations, mostly at background sites. Secondly, there appeared to be no real commitment on behalf of Government to secure car-free cities and locally-managed public transport systems. The policy of bus deregulation had been left largely to market determination.

The first step was to convince the local council that traffic pollution was a priority. This presented difficulties because there was no money to fund the initial monitoring. The environmental health officers decided to enter the barter economy. They located a reputable company which was just starting to enter the local authority monitoring market. In return for a free six-months loan of equipment, the environmental health officers gave the company a prime city centre site plus a place in their forward plan to develop a European initiative to highlight the above concerns.

Within six months, thanks to the results of the monitoring, the local council was convinced that they did have a traffic pollution problem and to their credit they gave full backing under their discretionary powers to move forward with the Airwatch Partnership Project. The main partners in the project are set out below in *Figure 8.1*.

Although it is still in its initial stages the partnership is already bearing fruit. Bonn is a car-free city, Lieden has developed a theoretical model of pollution forecasts, Grenoble has developed to a high degree central and local planning and Oxford has its park and ride. All these things are being shared with great benefit as is the local research on health and traffic. The point for health promotion practi-

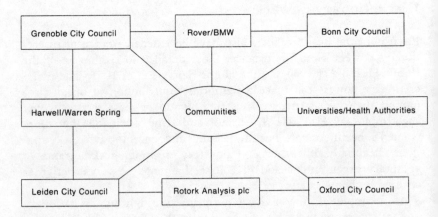

Figure 8.1   *Partners in the 'Airwatch Partnership Project'*

tioners is that the environmental health discretionary powers of local authorities can contribute to promoting health in a very real way.

Campaigns and projects

It is, perhaps, helpful in the context of this book to look at a number of local campaigns and projects where environmental health officers work in health promotion partnership with the health authority, commerce and industry.

Restaurants, cafes and hotels are regularly inspected by EHOs under the Food Safety Act and these officers are therefore in a strong position to encourage the statutory minimum standards. The Health Education Authority's Heartbeat Award scheme introduced jointly by the HEA and individual local authorities has provided a means for promoting and establishing healthy eating options and no-smoking areas in catering premises.

Some local authorities have gone further and established their own food awards for the catering industry which enhance the *Heartbeat* standard, and encourage additional health facilities such as baby-changing accommodation and provision of non-alcoholic drinks.

Commercial premises (other than catering premises) can also be encouraged in a similar fashion. One local authority introduced jointly with their health authority a health award. In order to attain the award, a company must comply completely with the Health and Safety at Work Act, and in addition commit itself to three approved *green* policies and three approved healthy lifestyle policies.

By setting up a good landlord or (to be politically correct) good *landpersons* award, a number of local authorities are promoting health by encouraging landpersons to see their business as a positive health contribution to the local community.

Participation in local campaigns and projects are laudable, but they are more effective when interacting with a national campaign. Such central organisations as the Health Education Authority or the Department of Health can set the national agenda by getting media coverage and high profile national figures. They can also provide expertise to give a campaign firm direction. Add to this the local authority's local network and there's productive synergy.

Local authorities through their EHOs can make important contributions to health promotion. Since 1974 when the medical officer was relocated in the health authority, the EHO has been seen as the local authority's lead officer on health matters. However, it is now recognised that to effectively promote health, professionals need to work on a collaborative basis, rather than as independent experts. Health is indeed everybody's business and if anyone should lead, it should be the community. It is now acknowledged that local government departments such as personnel education, social services and leisure also have key roles in the health promotion scenario. What parts they have to play will be discussed later in this book.

References

Bassett (1991). *Clay's Handbook of Environmental Health.* London: Chapman & Hall.

Department of Health (1992). *The Health of the Nation.* London: HMSO.

Institute of Environmental Health Officers (1993). *Guidance to Local Authorities on Smoking Policies.* London: IEHO.

Standing Conference on Public Health (1994). *A National Strategy for Housing.* London: SCPH.

Tones, K. (1990). Why theorise: ideology in health education. *Health Education Journal, 49,* 1.

9 *Promoting health through social services*

Linda Jones and Jon Bloomfield

Social services departments in the UK have a current workforce of over 306 000 and an annual budget in excess of £5000 million. In England alone, they provide care and support for around 55 000 children in local authority homes each year and for another 41 000 children who are on Child Protection Registers. In 1992, a total of 106 200 people, including the elderly, those with physical disabilities, learning disabilities and mental health problems were being supported by social services in local authority, voluntary or private residential homes (Central Statistical Office, 1994). Since 1993, the new arrangements for residential care under the National Health Service and Community Care Act (1990) mean that many more residents in voluntary and private homes have become the concern of social services departments. In addition, many thousands of families are visited by social workers each year and over 500 000 older and disabled people receive domiciliary services such as home help or meals-on-wheels.

This breadth of provision, delivered in a range of intimate and formal settings, indicates that social services may have considerable potential to promote people's health. In looking at their role, however, it is important to start off with an explicit recognition of their limitations. Unlike schools or GPs, these departments are not universal providers of services; the majority of citizens go through life without direct contact with them. Social services could not be expected to provide mass health promotion in the way that primary health care might aim to do. But, since they work with many of the most vulnerable, frail and socially disadvantaged people in society, they have a potentially strategic role in any overall health promotion strategy.

Many of the goals established for health promotion by the Ottawa Charter (WHO, 1986) are relevant to the work of social services. The Charter emphasises the need to create supportive environments, strengthen community action and develop personal skills, so that people have the resources to influence and improve their health. The Health of the Nation strategy (Department of Health, 1992) acknowledged the significance of 'healthy surroundings' and 'decent local environment and housing conditions' in improving health, noting that agencies outside the health sector, such as local authorities, had an important role to play.

In this chapter, we will argue that social services already engage in broad health promotion activity by protecting their clients and working to develop their skills for living. Beyond this, however, there is scope for a more comprehensive strategy for health promotion to be developed. The focus of this should be threefold: prevention, and intervening earlier to avoid crisis; health education, by offering appropriate information and support to clients; and helping to build healthy alliances which acknowledge the interrelatedness of social and health care goals. After discussing the current focus of social services we will draw attention to opportunities and new initiatives, and consider how such a strategy might be developed with different client groups.

The current focus of social services departments

In spite of increasing interest in prevention and health promotion there has been growing pressure on social service departments in recent years to concentrate their efforts and resources at the more intensive end of the care spectrum. Several important factors have influenced this development. Firstly, growing demand for services has outstripped the supply of resources. This is most evident with the rising population of the frail elderly. Secondly, growing social inequality and unemployment in the 1980s hit hardest at the bottom 20 per cent of the population (Central Statistical Office, 1994). As families find it more difficult to cope, so the workload of social services increases. Thirdly, there has been upheaval associated with restructuring of services, notably within social services departments themselves as they reorganise into commissioner and provider wings. National Health Service reforms have increased demand for social services. For example, the dramatic fall in the number of long-stay hospital geriatric beds is having a profound impact upon the type of home care services which are required.

Fourthly, specific Government legislation, such as the Mental Health Act 1983 and the Children Act 1989, and their sometimes legalistic and defensive interpretations by social services, have led to an over-concentration on those deemed to be most at risk, particularly children. Media coverage of child abuse, highlighting shortcomings within social work, has exacerbated its general defensiveness and thereby contributed to a major shift in focus away from general preventive work with families. At times there has seemed to be an almost exclusive concentration on protection (Audit Commission, 1994).

These trends have been abetted by a drive to professionalisation within departments, along with erratic attempts at improved management. One important and unforeseen consequence has been that basic caring and helping tasks have been downgraded.

A shift towards prevention?

If a defensive culture remains, there is little chance of health promotion work gaining ground within social service departments. However, there are signs of a change in emphasis in some authorities which could align social services more closely with health promotion objectives. The Social Services Inspectorate are now becoming aware of the dangers for children and families of this over concentration on the 'heavy end' of the service, and have called for a shift in emphasis towards the preventative and family support aspects of the Children Act. Similarly, moves to develop a more generally preventive social work practice are evident in the attempts to link up social workers directly with GPs and primary health care teams. The hospital social worker's central role in assessing the needs of patients before discharge may provide new opportunities. Such moves could help to give a broader and more preventive focus to social work services.

The case for prevention in social care is analogous to that in health care, and is already being applied in the area of community care. The basic premise of community care is that it can be more effective and less expensive to support people in their own homes or in non-institutional settings which maintain their independence for as long as possible (Department of Health, 1989). In social work with children and families this could translate into more, but relatively less expensive, systems for family support leading to fewer family breakdowns and, in the long run, to less need for very expensive interventions and institutional care.

The health categorisation of primary, secondary and tertiary prevention provides a useful starting point for conceptualising these social care interventions (Parker, 1980; Hardiker *et al.*, 1991). Fuller (1992) argues that primary prevention in social work, prominent in the community development projects of the 1960s and characterised as 'influencing the social-structural origins of personal troubles,...' largely belongs in the category of abandoned ambitions. A more limited doctrine of primary prevention would focus on strategies to improve the parenting capacities of those under stress, or to influence local authorities to provide more services to those at risk to enhance their choices and quality of life. Alongside this must be placed the goals of secondary prevention – to offer services to those experiencing difficulties but not yet in crisis – and tertiary prevention

– to mitigate the damaging effects of breakdown. In practice, however, these neat divisions break down and clients may be at different stages in their relationships with different agencies (Hardiker *et al.*, 1991).

Preventive work with children and families

What scope is there for prevention – primary, secondary or tertiary – with children and families? Here the key to change is the priorities of social work services. Are they going to be almost entirely focused on child protection, investigating cases of physical and sexual abuse, or can these protective services be complemented and underpinned by a broader network of services which support families in trouble before breakdown and violence occurs? For prevention to succeed, social services must offer support and advice to these families; for example, to modify an unruly child's behaviour, to stimulate networks of support and self-reliance within these communities, to offer some simple practical help such as occasional respite during a family crisis, some counselling, or simply a way through the benefits maze.

The case for prevention

A move to focus significant, even if limited, resources on prevention would not only lead to more effective social work but would also be an important step towards promoting health. Such help could not only reduce stress levels in families, violence and family breakdown, but also the numbers of mothers visiting GPs for depression and the problems being stored up for future generations by children experiencing disturbed childhoods. Research by Ruth Gardner of the Children's Society indicates that, at present, preventive work suffers from a lack of communication and coordination between agencies as compared with child protection (Cervi, 1994). The Children Act may have reduced the access of deprived families to social services, so that problems are getting picked up later. Jane Aldgate, monitoring section 17 of the Children Act for the Department of Health, comments that 'families with a great deal of deprivation, which are classic families which social services traditionally helped, are getting less services' (quoted in Cervi, 1994, p. 17).

The Audit Commission report (1994) calls for a shift to redirect resources towards prevention, through provisions such as playgroups, community support and family centres, and this is supported by senior Department of Health officer, Wendy Rose (cited in Stone, 1994, p. 16):

It is not acceptable nor consistent with the Children Act philosophy for the gateway to family support services to be closed until the problem is presented in terms of child protection... The primary focus of a social services department is not to find out whether a child has been abused or a criminal offence has occurred. Have we strayed from the notion of a social worker making inquiries and visiting a family at home to see if she or he can be helpful?

One criticism of prevention concerns the difficulty of evaluating it, but research on the Mobile Action Resource Service (MARS) project in Dundee, managed by Barnados and Tayside Regional Council, indicates that 'secondary prevention' strategies can be effective in preventing children entering care (Fuller, 1992). The project reported on 34 cases and had a success rate of 75 per cent in relation to the primary objective – keeping children out of care. This was tested through a *predictor test*; asking a panel of five social workers to study six of the cases and predict outcomes. In all these cases their predictions were more gloomy than the actual outcome, and their assessments indicate that the MARS project had played a major role in preventing family crisis and disintegration.

Day care and residential services

One important component of this preventive family support work focuses on the day care services which social services can either provide or arrange. Where they run their own nurseries, these could also be a base for local mothers' groups, or for the health visitor to run regular clinics. Health education advice might be offered where appropriate; for example, the importance of diet could be stressed when day care officers register childminders and when they visit them.

There may be opportunities for broader interventions to promote health as well. Links could be established by day care officers between nursery schools and childminders, for example, so that parents with a part-time nursery school place can make easy arrangements for childminding. After all, enabling people in low-income households to work is crucial to improving the health of both themselves and their children.

In addition, social services departments have a particular responsibility and a unique opportunity to promote the health of children within their own residential homes. These children are often amongst the most damaged and vulnerable of their generation, survivors of family breakdown, physical violence and sexual abuse. On occasion, they are targeted by those eager to make new recruits to the world of prostitution; hence the key importance of specific sexual health programmes for all children's homes. Given the sensitivity of these issues, for instance giving contraceptive advice to under-16 year olds, and the tendency of the press to sensationalise, this is an area where the closest cooperation with local health authorities and their health promotion teams is particularly important. Several social services departments have undertaken joint work with district health authorities and it is undoubtedly an area which would repay attention across all departments.

Sexual health advice is a top priority but it is only part of a wider possible health education strategy. Department of Health (1994) guidelines on smoking and alcohol consumption in residential homes now advise that no child under 16 years should smoke, that staff should not smoke in front of children and that they and visitors should only smoke in a designated smoking room. Although desirable in health education terms, this could add to problems of control in residential homes, where cigarettes have become part of a 'reward system' (Siddall, 1994). Teenage smokers with challenging behaviour will find it even harder to cope, and smoking could be driven underground. A more innovative approach to changing smoking behaviour might be to offer clients (and workers) the type of individual-focused assessment and intensive, continuing support that has proved successful with some hospital patients (Macleod Clark *et al.*, 1990).

Underpinning health education, there needs to be a broader strategic approach to health promotion. For example, Boulton (1993) pointed out that people leaving local authority care constitute one of the groups most likely to become homeless. Most young people are taught few skills for independent living; they find it difficult to cook, budget or manage the benefits system. Residential homes may teach skills for group living, but they also encourage young people to rely on authority to sort out problems. Moreover, local authority care ends abruptly when young people are eighteen. A policy of prevention, with more gradual withdrawal of support, intensive 'pre-release' programmes of health and social education and trial 'living alone' experiments, could enhance the independence and well-being of these young people.

People with special needs

Most aspects of social services work relating to people with special needs have health promotion dimensions. For instance, the day-care services provided for people with physical or learning disabilities and those with mental health problems sustain the general welfare and well-being of users, and offer a vital break for carers from often onerous care responsibilities. The assessment of needs and provision for equipment and adaptations to enable people to carry on living in their own homes is a vital service benefiting tens of thousands of people each year.

In many authorities there is scope for significant improvements in the way this assessment and adaptation work is handled, and in liaison between different council departments and outside agencies. The disability charity RADAR, in a recent survey, found delays in providing home adaptations to be the main cause of complaint to local authorities (Ivory, 1993). An underlying influence is lack of resources; all departments are finding that reductions in central government housing allocations mean that the sums available for major adaptations via the Disabled Facilities Grant are increasingly limited. Lack of resources influences assessment as well. Since departments are bound under law to provide the full range of resources once needs are demonstrated, social workers are more likely to make a conservative estimate of need in case they are unable to meet it.

The health dimension is probably most evident in the arena of mental health. Here social work has a key role in counselling, support and advice, helping citizens to overcome specific mental health problems and arranging for specific medical and nursing services where needed. The creation of a new fund, the Mental Illness Specific Grant, has been an important if limited step. Despite its short-term character and the requirement for local authorities to find 30 per cent of the funding for each scheme, it has been one of the few pieces of genuinely new money which has been made available for additional community care responsibilities. Many local authorities have sought to use this money to provide supported accommodation for people with mental health problems and to extend both the range and opening times of day services.

Services for elderly people

Social services departments have direct contact with many thousands of older people through home care and meals-on-wheels services. Whether these services are directly provided or arranged on a contract basis by a voluntary agency or a private firm there are real opportunities for departments to ensure that there is a health dimension to this work. Home carers have access to thousands of elderly people each week and often have considerable (unused) knowledge and understanding of the needs of their clients (Evers *et al.*, 1994). They could not only offer information, for example on winter warmth campaigns, domestic accidents, and access to services, but also provide much more of a link between clients and health and social services professionals. The shift from home help, with its emphasis on cleaning and mechanical tasks, to home care, with its focus on personal as well as home care, is vital here (Tinker, 1990). But there is evidence that local authorities are so busy attempting to meet the rising demands for home care that they do not sufficiently evaluate their provision (Hoyes *et al.*, 1994). Althea Tinker (1990, p. 56) comments that:

> the kinds of services which will be wanted [in future] are those which are individually tailored to needs. Surveys of nearly every service show that there are people receiving it who neither need it nor want it.

A health promotion approach might target home care organisers, who currently have little support and low professional qualifications (Department of Health and Social Security, 1986), so that their role in home care (including, possibly, health advice) could be extended. Training and support for informal carers would also feature on this agenda. Over six million people are currently caring for a relative or friend at home (Office of Population Censuses and Surveys, 1990) and recent reports have highlighted carers' needs for practical as well as emotional support (Bibbings, 1994). One long-term carer commented that 'caring can damage your health' (Leventon, 1990) and recent reports have highlighted the need for advice on lifting techniques, first aid and diet.

Resource problems threaten to undermine domiciliary services. As local authority grants from central government are squeezed, some social services departments are moving towards means-testing (Rickford, 1994). Some older and disabled people will be able to pay, but for others the fear of large bills for services such as laundry or extra heating and the stigma of means-testing may well deter them from applying for help. More fundamentally, such policies signal a reluctant response by local authorities to central government's tacit redrawing of the boundaries between health and social care. Whereas patients in long-stay hospitals had such services provided free under the National Health Service, people in their own homes are now being asked to pay. This puts a policy of prevention and community care at risk; the effects of means-testing could well be higher admission rates to hospitals and residential care in the longer term.

Interagency working

There are also organisational changes which will improve interagency cooperation and the capacity of departments to deliver health gains. A recent study, for example, has highlighted the crucial role of housing across the whole of community care policy and the relative lack of attention paid to it at the planning stage (Arnold *et al.*, 1993). Clearly, it is important that social services departments link closely with their counterparts in housing so that vulnerable groups, such as teenagers leaving local authority care, are given active consideration on housing department waiting lists.

There is also considerable scope for social services staff to liaise and network more effectively with doctors and community health staff in primary health care teams, an outcome probably best achieved by attaching social workers to general practices. This would help not just to break down professional barriers, but would also ease access to services for clients and encourage the development of more seamless services. At present there is evidence that community care implementation is patchy, carers and users are unenthusiastic and general practitioners are the weakest link – 'poorly involved and ill-informed' (Henwood, 1994). It is information, advice and support from social services that will largely change these views and help to bring family doctors *on board*.

Beyond this, Dalley (1993) draws attention to the health work–social work divide, arguing that professional training and occupational culture imbue these services with attitudes and values which are difficult to change. Experience of professional working reinforces tribal loyalties and, when hard decisions have to be made, workers split along specialist professional lines. If health and social services are to work together to meet the client's health promotion needs, then such cleavages need to be recognised and tackled.

Recently, there has been evidence of much closer cooperation between the health and social services. There is increasing liaison over community care planning and, although social services were directed to consult rather than to involve health authorities in the planning stage, many departments have moved beyond this towards genuine interagency working (Giraud-Saunders, 1994). In Bromley, for example, joint commissioning began in 1991 after a history of joint working in the community care area and the longer-term aim is to focus on 'joint action to influence the health and quality of life for all Bromley residents' (Standish *et al.*, 1994). In the 1990s, as health and social services joint commissioning expands, there will be increasing opportunities for health promotion to move up the agenda of social services departments.

It is hoped that this chapter has sparked a number of ideas of possible ways forward for local authority social services departments. Some professionals will throw their hands up in horror and say it is naive to imagine that at a time of sharp cut backs and retrenchment, social services can take on a broader brief. It is undeniable that all the frontline services are under pressure. But the future of social services lies, above all, in their ability to respond to a broad range of social problems and to provide genuine practical help to families and citizens in need. And that broader prospective has a health dimension, both by providing care and support and by enabling and encouraging self-reliance. It is a route that they should be encouraged to follow, no matter how hard pressed social services departments become.

References

Audit Commission (1994). *The Community Revolution: Personal Social Services and Community Care*. London, HMSO.

Bibbings, A. (1994). Carers and professionals – the carer's viewpoint. In A. Leathard (ed.), *Going Inter-Professional*, pp. 158–171. London: Routledge.

Boulton, I. (1993). Youth homelessness and health care. In K. Fisher & J. Collins (eds), *Homelessness and Health Care*, pp. 140–153. London: Longman.

Arnold, P., Bochel, H., Brochurst, S. & Page, D. (1993). *Community Care: The Housing Dimension*. London: Community Care/Joseph Rowntree Foundation.

Central Statistical Office (1994). *Social Trends*, vol. 24. London: HMSO.

Cervi, R. (1994). Real lives. *Community Care* (20 January), 16–17.

Dalley, G. (1993). Professional ideology or organisational tribalism? The health work–social work divide. In J. Walmsley, J. Reynolds, P. Shakespeare & R. Wolfe (eds), *Health, Welfare and Practice*. London, Sage.

Department of Health (1989). *Caring For People*, Cmd. 849. London: HMSO.

Department of Health (1990). *National Health Service and Community Care Act*. London: HMSO.

Department of Health (1992). *The Health of the Nation*. London: HMSO.

Department of Health (1994). *Guidelines on Smoking and Alcohol Consumption in Residential Care Establishments*. London: HMSO.

Department of Health & Social Security (1986). Neighbourhood nursing: a focus for care. Cumberledge Committee Report. London: HMSO.

Evers, H., Cameron, E. & Badger, F. (1994). Inter-professional work with old and disabled people. In A. Leathard (ed.), *Going Inter-Professional*, pp. 143–157. London: Routledge.

Fuller, R. (1992). *In Search of Prevention*. Aldershot: Avebury.

Giraud-Saunders, A. (1994). New patterns of care. *Health Service Journal* (13 October), 32–33.

Hardiker, P., Exton, K. & Barker, M. (1991). *Policies and Practice in Preventive Child Care*. Aldershot: Avebury.

Henwood, M. (1994). *Fit For Change? Snapshots of the Community Care Reforms One Year On*. London: King's Fund/Nuffield Institute.

Hoyes, L., Lart, R., Means, R. & Taylor, M. (1994). *Community Care in Transition*. London: Community Care/Joseph Rowntree Foundation.

Ivory, M. (1993). Assessing the waiting game. *Community Care*, 23 September.

Leventon, S. (1990). The realities of caring: an inside view. In P. Carter et al. (eds), *Social Work and Social Welfare*, pp. 172–183. Buckingham: Open University Press.

Macleod Clark, J., Kendall, S. and Haverty, S. (1990). Helping people to stop smoking: a study of the nurse's role. *Journal of Advanced Nursing*, *15*, 3, 357–63.

Macleod Clark, J. & Latter, S. (1992). Factors influencing nurses' health education and health promotion practice in acute ward areas. In J. Wilson-Barnett & J. Macleod Clark (eds), *Research in Health Promotion and Nursing*, pp. 61–71. London: Macmillan.

Office of Population Censuses and Surveys (1990). *General Household Survey*. London: OPCS.

Parker, R. A. (ed.) (1980). *Caring for Separated Children*. London: Macmillan.

Rickford, F. (1994). Elderly shocked by means testing. *Community Care*, 6–10 October.

Siddall, R. (1994). Fag end. *Community Care* (24 February), 16–17.

Standish, S., Perry, C. & Palk, N. (1994). Scoring doubles. *Health Service Journal* (15 September), 26–27.

Stone, K. (1994). The 'at risk' trap. *Community Care* (10–16 November), 16–17.

Tinker, A. (1990). Planning for a new generation of older people. In P. Carter et al. (eds), *Social Work and Social Welfare*, pp. 54–63. Buckingham: Open University Press.

World Health Organisation (1986). *The Ottawa Charter*. Ottawa: WHO.

10 *Health promotion through leisure services*

Robin Ireland

This chapter concentrates on the work of local authority leisure services departments. It begins by giving an impression of the national picture and social and economic factors, before considering the work of the local authority itself. Some time will be spent considering the implications of compulsory competitive tendering (CCT), before looking at issues surrounding past and present collaborations between health promotion and leisure professionals.

The national picture

Great Britain has never had a single national government agency responsible for the promotion of exercise and fitness. The Sports Council has seen its responsibility as the promotion and organisation of sport, whereas the Health Education Authority has considered healthy lifestyles, but with little focus on exercise. The Allied Dunbar National Fitness Survey (ADNFS), which published its findings in 1992, was the most important collaborative effort around physical activity for many years and was the largest survey of its kind in the world. Its findings are disturbing. Whilst 80 per cent of both women and men believed themselves to be fit, in fact only 30 per cent of men and 20 per cent of women take sufficient exercise to achieve a health benefit; that is, levels of activity accepted as offering some protection against coronary heart disease and conferring a wide range of other health and functional benefits.

Unfortunately, the role of the Sports Council has been unclear under the Conservative Government, spending time in the Department of Education and the Department of Environment before reaching its present home in the Department of National Heritage. The advent of the National Lottery may see the Sports Council becoming mainly a funding organisation, in addition to its two other principal areas of work with young people and the development of performance and excellence in sport. The days of the promotion of mass participation and the egalitarian 'Sport for All' appear to have long gone. The

Minister of Sport in 1994 was quoted as saying 'When I talk about sport in schools I do not mean step aerobics, going for country walks ... I want team games properly organised – competitive team games' (as quoted in *The Guardian*, 28 January 1994).

The Department of Health, through the Health Education Authority, has moved closer towards a clearer objective of promoting physical activity. After *The Health of the Nation* failed to define targets for physical activity as a part of the Coronary Heart Disease and Stroke Key Area, a Physical Activity Task Force was set up which publicised its findings in early 1995. Although no targets have been determined, the messages are clearer than before; to increase the proportion of men and women taking moderate and vigorous intensity physical activity. A national campaign to encourage people to take more physical activity is being launched in 1995 with a single message that is broadly applicable to the majority of the population: 'Take 30 minutes of moderate physical activity, such as a sustained brisk walk, on at least five days of the week.'

Although this chapter takes as its concern the promotion of physical activity amongst the population as a whole, it is worth noting that several developments have taken place in recent years to encourage young people to take more exercise. For example, changes in the national curriculum, which include an entitlement for all young people to a physical education. The Education Reform Acts of 1986 and 1988, and local management of schools, are influencing the extent to which school facilities are made available to the local community. Major projects such as the Happy Hearts Project (University of Hull), the Health and Physical Education Project (Loughborough University) and Active Lifestyles (a Sports Council National Demonstration Project in Coventry), have promoted physical activity amongst school-aged children.

Health promotion and sports development

The Sports Council developed a number of National Demonstration Projects in the 1980s in association with a variety of organisations (the Sports Council, 1991). The aim was to promote mass participation through establishing new partnerships and developing new ways of working with different groups. The conclusions drawn from these projects have helped to inform the work of the Sports Council in the 1990s.

The idea of a sports development continuum has long been a central tenet to current thinking regarding the development of individuals and organisations in maximising their sporting potential. In the model illustrated (*Figure 10.1*), McDonald and Tungatt (1992)

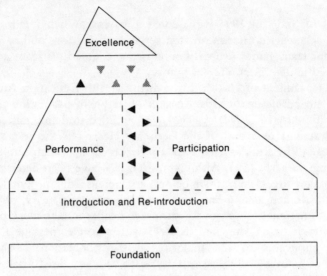

Source: McDonald and Tungatt (1992). Reproduced with permission of the Sports Council and the authors

Figure 10.1   *Sports development model*

suggest that there are four areas of involvement: firstly, *foundation* is defined as the acquisition of basic skills; secondly, *participation* is taking part in defined activities for recreational purposes; thirdly, *performance* is the process of getting better at a particular activity; and finally, *excellence* is the achievement of a national standard according to absolute criteria. Health promotion can be seen as having a positive role in the foundation and participation stages. The foundation stage can be linked to the population as a whole, rather than limiting it to those of primary school age only. Health providers can be seen to encourage the sedentary majority of the British population to take up physical activity and, for some, to move into the sports development continuum and to the range of opportunities within it.

Leisure provision

Local authorities have traditionally been major providers and operators of sports facilities. Unlike the private sector, they have been able to pursue broad objectives such as health promotion or the alleviation of social deprivation. Local authorities in this country have been under at least as much pressure as the National Health Service in recent years. The provision of leisure services is not a statutory requirement of local government unlike education and social services. Leisure departments may be found in various guises across Britain:

education, arts and leisure, as well as tourism, may all be within the department which organises leisure if, indeed, leisure provision exists. Sports development sections, within recreation and leisure departments, which had flourished under the Sports Council's Sport for All policy have been severely cut back in the early 1990s, and this process is likely to continue as budgets are rigorously pruned.

Leisure provision has been divided into client and contractor services, broadly mirroring the purchaser and provider organisation within the NHS. Compulsory competitive tendering for local government services was introduced as a part of the Local Government Acts of 1980 and 1988, and was extended to sport and leisure management in 1988. Under the Act, if local authorities wanted their own direct service organisation (DSO) to bid, they were required to tender competitively for the management functions of a range of sport and leisure facilities.

In practice, the management of very few leisure centres was taken on by private contractors. The Sports Council report that 84 per cent of contracts were won by DSOs (the Sports Council, 1993). However, the pressure on leisure departments was considerable as officers struggled to cope with the demands and pressures of a new market. Contracts were financial rather than social, and sports development led and contained little if any specifications regarding socially and economically disadvantaged groups. This has led to barriers to sports development policies attracting wider sections of the community into using local facilities and taking part in sport.

The potential for alliances

As local authority leisure services battle with a new round of tenders and contracts, an opportunity arises to work with health authority purchasers to provide health promotion services for their communities. Health differences have long been shown to reflect socioeconomic status (Townsend *et al.*, 1992), and current health strategies seek to take into account health imbalances in urban and rural areas (North West Council for Sport and Recreation, 1994; North West Regional Health Authority, 1994a,b). The remainder of this chapter focuses on a number of key areas which offer possibilities for leisure and health providers working together.

Leisure providers are fast becoming aware of the importance of the health factor in leisure provision. Posts currently available for leisure services staff (as advertised in the Institute of Leisure and Amenity Management Appointments service) include an Exercise and Health Development Officer (funded with a health purchaser to develop long-term participation in exercise); an Exercise Development Officer (funded with a health promotion agency to establish a GP referral scheme); and a Health and Recreation Coordinator (working at a sports centre to supervise a new cardiovascular suite). These new posts reflect the range of alliances and activities now available within health and leisure agencies.

District sport and recreation strategies

The Sports Council has been encouraging local authorities to adopt a strategic approach to the planning and development of leisure services (the Sports Council, 1991). The preparation of district sport and recreation strategies should include a period of consultation with the local community and with a number of public sector and voluntary organisations. Health purchasers must ensure that their message is clearly understood by local authorities in terms of increasing the opportunities for physical activity for all sectors of the community. Health authorities may combine with local authorities in the development of exercise strategies. Whichever approach is adopted, a clear framework should be established to develop local targets for participation and to establish contracting mechanisms.

These targets may not simply be about the provision of leisure facilities, but may involve the safe use of parks, environmental improvements to public rights of way in the countryside, the cleaning up of seashores, river and canal banks. The Trans-Pennine Trail, a long-distance path from coast to coast, providing opportunities for runners, walkers, cyclists and horse riders, is an excellent example of agencies working together to create recreational and environmental benefits. Thirty local authorities and the Countryside Commission are cooperating to construct, promote, maintain and manage the Trail.

Leisure facilities

The Sports Council has established that less than half of all local authorities in England (34 per cent) and Scotland (36 per cent) have a sport and recreation strategy. At the same time, it has recognised that the introduction of competitive tendering has made the role of local authorities in the development of Sport for All even more important (the Sports Council, 1993). As the Sports Council argues, developing sport and recreation as part of a local authority's leisure strategy brings a number of benefits. Some of these apply equally to health service providers, such as the development of the individual; community development; health improvements; economic improvements; improving the quality of life; and relief of social deprivation (the Sports Council, 1994).

By developing strategic objectives for inclusion in local authority leisure management specifications, health authorities can play a key role in supporting Sport for All policies. Examples include the provision of Leisure Cards to enable people on low incomes to receive price reductions and priority booking benefits. Computerised registration and leisure-card schemes can also enable a leisure-centre manager to monitor usage by different parts of the community and to gauge the extent, for example, that women, disabled and black people use a facility. Positive action, such as women-only sessions with crèche facilities, can be taken to encourage wider usage and target non-participants. Programmes such as Sandwell Asian Women's Exercise and Recreational Activities (SAWERA), have aimed to increase opportunities for participation in sport and recreation by Asian women.

Many local authority leisure centres now have cardiovascular fitness suites as managers seek to attract new customers. These suites have often replaced old-fashioned weights rooms. The clientele have also changed, encouraging a new range of participants, more health conscious and less interested in body building. These facilities offer excellent opportunities for health workers to refer their patients. These may be referrals from primary care, to increase exercise levels in order to reduce the risk of coronary heart disease and to lose weight, or as secondary care referrals from hospitals (for example, the Wear Fit cardiac rehabilitation programme in south and west Durham) or to physiotherapists for rehabilitation after injuries or operations.

There are also examples of providing transport for people to leisure facilities where public transport is inadequate (such as the Stockport Swimbus scheme). There is an opportunity here for health authorities to make alliances with local authorities to widen the scope for health promotion and healthcare (Chalmers, 1993). The National Health Service should be prepared to subsidise exercise facilities in return for increasing the physical activity levels of target populations.

Physical activity promotion in primary health care

Leisure centres now frequently offer a referral point for primary health care workers who wish to give their patients an exercise prescription. The link between diagnostic medical services and leisure provision can be traced back to the Peckham Health Centre in the 1920s and 1930s (Scott-Samuel, 1990). This pioneering health centre had consulting rooms, a gymnasium and swimming pool within the same building. Subsequent projects such as the Health and Recreation Team in Liverpool (the Sports Council, 1987), took referrals from health workers and gave patients a series of exercise options. More recently still, Hailsham Lagoon's Oasis programme has received a great deal of publicity because of its success in taking referrals from local doctors to the Lagoon Leisure Centre.

Primary health care workers hold a unique position in identifying and influencing those patients who may best benefit from increased physical activity. A report commissioned by the Health Education Authority (Biddle *et al.*, 1994) found at least 121 primary health care schemes promoting physical activity in England. However, their research also shows that schemes only reach a very small proportion of the patient base. Care must be taken in setting up protocols for such schemes, so that GPs, Family Health Services Authorities and leisure services staff, are clear about their objectives. For example GPs may wish to refer patients who have multiple risk factors (hypertension and obesity for instance) from coronary heart disease, whilst leisure centre managers may simply have fastened onto an idea which they hope will help to fill their off-peak time.

The patients who are referred in the above situation may well be the people least likely to use a leisure centre in other circumstances, and may well be alienated from the scheme immediately. It is important to consider the type of activities offered at the recreational facility and the staff employed to run them in these circumstances. Health authorities have assisted in a number of examples to help finance Health and Fitness Coordinators who receive the referrals direct from the GPs. A contribution may also be made to the cost of activities at a leisure centre.

There are a number of training courses in lifestyle health education skills such as the 'Look After Yourself' programme and 'Helping People Change'. These types of courses provide an opportunity for leisure centre staff to consider an individual's lifestyle development and the personal needs of their customers. It may well be necessary to set up special sessions for the referrals which include exercise to music and simple circuit training. Biddle *et al.* (*ibid*) describe other types of physical activity promotion in primary health care which are all worth investigating, including the solitary but enthusiastic GP, the practice-based exercise clinic, a health centre–community approach and GP referrals to private health clubs.

A last comment is necessary about the most common type of referral, namely GP to leisure centre. If leisure centres are to be seen as health promoting centres, they will need to develop smoking, alcohol and nutrition policies. There is no reason why local authority sports centres cannot follow the example set by private health clubs and offer users healthy snacks in place of junk food, and still meet financial targets.

Promoting sport for all

Health services have an important role to play in helping to make healthier lifestyles more accessible to the general public. This does not need to be an approach where an individual is made to feel guilty about their lifestyle, whilst ignoring environmental and economic factors such as housing and employment status. Physical activity can be a positive choice for the majority. The North West Regional Health Authority (and formerly Mersey Regional Health Authority) has taken a lead in recent years in both mass fitness testing and developing mass participation exercise activities. Events such as the North West Regional Health Corporate Series, seven five-kilometre runs and walks across the north west of England, have helped to promote health and fitness in the workplace, as well as developing closer ties between health and leisure agencies. Health Start, a six-week lifestyles festival and a part of the Health at Work in the NHS initiative, will further help to promote the benefits of physical activity to NHS staff and the public as a whole in the north west.

Health has a crucial role in making sport itself more welcoming to prospective participants. The very term 'sport' has served to alienate the majority of the British population. Many people's memory of taking part in sport at school is of a competitive environment, rather like a number of Conservative Ministers of Sport would appear to support, where the physically inarticulate are metaphorically and physically exiled to the sidelines. This is not in any way arguing that there is no place for competition, but that this should be a matter of choice. Each individual should have the opportunity to take part in their chosen physical activity at the most appropriate level. That level may be determined by how far an individual wishes to progress in their particular sport or form of exercise, or by the limits to their ability. The sports development model discussed earlier shows how individuals are able to progress from foundation to participation level. Some will continue on to performance and the smallest group of all will progress on to excellence. The key seems to me to be in providing that potential journey for all parts of the community, black and white, female and male, disabled and non-disabled, old and young. Health providers have an opportunity to work with and encourage local authority leisure providers to ensure that their facilities and sports are open to all and not simply the athletically gifted, self confident, fitness motivated sections of our community.

References

Activity and Health Research (1992). *Allied Dunbar National Fitness Survey:*

114   *Robin Ireland*

Main Findings. London: the Sports Council and the Health Education Authority.

Ashton, J. & Seymour, H. (1990). *The New Public Health.* Buckingham: Open University Press.

The Audit Commission (1990). *Local Authority Support for Sport: A Management Handbook.* London: HMSO.

The Audit Commission (1989). *Sport for Whom? Clarifying the Local Authority Role in Sport and Recreation.* London: HMSO.

Biddle, S., Fox, K. & Edmunds, L. (1994). *Physical Activity Promotion in Primary Health Care in England: Final research project for Health Education Authority.* London: Health Education Authority.

Bowler, I. (1994). Activity alliances for health. *The Leisure Manager,* December 1994/January 1995.

Carroll, J. & Green, F. (1993). *Exercise on Prescription: A Report of the Pilot Scheme to Prescribe Exercise as part of a Coronary Heart Disease Prevention Programme.* Stockport: Leisure Services Division, Stockport MBC, Stockport Health Authorities.

Chalmers, F. (1993). Pulling together in King's Heath. *Healthlines,* 20 November. London: Health Education Authority.

Department of Health (1992). *The Health of the Nation: A Strategy for Health in England.* London: HMSO.

Drew, S. (1994). Exercise brings new life to Wirral. *Sportsnews.* Autumn 1994. Sports Council North West Region.

Health Education Authority (1990). *Take Heart: Good Practices in Coronary Heart Disease Prevention.* London: Health Education Authority.

Keele University (1994). Promoting physical activity through partnerships, unpublished paper.

McDonald, D. & Tungatt, M. (1992). *Community Development and Sport.* London: Community Development Foundation and the Sports Council.

North West Council for Sport and Recreation (1994). *Sign Up for Sport: The Regional Strategy for Sport and Recreation in the North West 1994–2000.* Manchester: North West Council for Sport and Recreation.

North West Regional Health Authority (1994a). *Patterns of Health: Improving Health in the North West.* Leeds: NHS Executive.

North West Regional Health Authority (1994b). *Strategic Statement: Improving Health in the North West.* Leeds: NHS Executive.

Scott-Samuel, A. (ed) (1990). *Total Participation, Total Health: Reinventing the Peckham Health Centre for the 1990s.* Edinburgh: Scottish Academic Press.

The Sports Council (1987). *Health and Recreation Team (HART) Mersey Regional Health Authority; Phase 2 Monitoring Report.* Manchester: The Sports Council.

The Sports Council (1991). *District Sport and Recreation Strategies: A Guide.* London: The Sports Council.

The Sports Council (1991). *National Demonstration Projects: Major Lessons and Issues for Sports Development.* London: The Sports Council.

The Sports Council (1993). *Compulsory Competitive Tendering for Sport and Leisure Management: National Information Survey Report.* London: The Sports Council.

The Sports Council (1993). *Young People and Sport: Policy and frameworks for Action.* London: The Sports Council.

The Sports Council (1994). *Developing Sport through CCT.* London: The Sports Council.

Torkildsen, G. (1983). *Leisure and Recreation Management*. London: E & F N Spon.

Townsend, P., Davidson, N. & Whitehead, M. (1992). *Inequalities in Health – The Black Report and the Health Divide*. London: Penguin.

Trades Union Congress (1982). *The Unequal Health of the Nation: A TUC Summary of the Black Report*. London: Trades Union Congress.

Education and youth organisations

11 The impact of recent government policy on the provision of health education in schools

Angela Scriven

Several years have passed since the government first proposed radical ideas for a major overhaul of the education system in England and Wales. These ideas were encapsulated into the Education Reform Act, ERA (Department for Education and Science, 1987). The implementation of the ERA has resulted in major changes to both the management of the education system and the curriculum of schools. This chapter assesses the implications of this, and other recent government policies, on the potential for teachers to provide effective school-based health education programmes and to form collaborative partnerships with external agencies in support of such initiatives.

Professional consensus on health education

There are a number of areas of professional consensus in relation to the current position of health education in schools. There is general agreement, for example, that schools are a key setting for the promotion of health (Department of Health, 1992; Denman, 1994; Naidoo and Wills, 1994). Downie *et al.* (1990) are not alone in expostulating a number of reasons in support of this claim. First, and in accordance with the preventive philosophy inherent in health promotion, it clearly makes more sense to encourage young people to adopt healthy lifestyles than to attempt to change unhealthy behaviour patterns in adulthood, particularly as evidence suggests that the risk factors for disease in adulthood often originate in early life. Secondly, and most importantly, a school provides an ideal environment for delivering a properly planned and coordinated programme of personal, social and health education to all children from the ages of 5 to 16.

Given these points, it is hardly surprising that a second area of general consensus concerning the health education curriculum in schools is that the years between the 1970s and 1990 proved to be a sustained period of growth and innovation. It is not the purpose of this chapter to give a potted history of the development of the subject, or indeed, to make a case for the continued need for health education in schools; there are good examples of this elsewhere. See, for example, Tones and Tilford (1990), Lewis (1993) and Emmett (1994). Let it suffice to say that by the early 1980s, research carried out by Southampton University for the Health Education Council (HEC) on a 12.5 per cent sample of all state schools in England and Wales indicated that 91 per cent of the sample were either providing health education or intending to do so (Williams and Roberts, 1985). A later study undertaken by Mori and commissioned by the successors of the HEC, The Health Education Authority, found that 77 per cent of primaries, 91 per cent of secondaries and 94 per cent of special schools either had a health education policy, or were planning to develop such a policy (MORI, 1989). It would appear, therefore, that by the late 1980s the need for, and commitment to, health education was demonstrated by its presence on the curriculum of most primary and secondary schools in the UK.

The effectiveness of this health education is not altogether clear. However, there is evidence to suggest that during this time there was considerable innovation taking place. Tones (1988), for example, discusses at some length the gradual move away from the medical model which dominated early health education programmes in schools, to a greater emphasis on values and attitudes and the importance of personal and social factors. This shift in focus and approach is demonstrated through the various programmes that became a feature of work in health education during this time. Leslie Button's (1984) *Developmental Group Work* and Hopson and Scally's (1981) *Lifeskills Teaching* although initially designed for youth-work settings and personal and social education programmes, respectively, were fundamental in influencing the move towards more experiential approaches in health education and, as a consequence, redefining the subject. Why then, after a period of rapid and inspired developments, have we seen increasing during the 1990s a more pessimistic outlook on the future of health education in schools? The prevailing view, as depicted in professional and academic journals, appears to be that the immediate future for health education is uncertain (Lewis, 1993; Emmett, 1994; Scriven, 1995). There is little doubt that the shift in mood from one of optimism to one of despondency has coincided with the implementation of the ERA. To understand what it is about the Act that has resulted in a perceived negative impact on the delivery of the health education curriculum, one must consider the key elements of the government's reforms.

The national curriculum and its impact on health education

The introduction of a national curriculum (NC) was seen as the central thrust of the ERA. The ten statutory core and foundation subjects, with associated assessment, apply throughout the years of schooling, from the ages of 5 to 16. Health education is not designated a statutory subject, but one of five cross curricular themes intended to be taught through the foundation subjects and through separate provision (National Curriculum Council (1990)). Initially, there was some criticism of the national curriculum by those with a professional interest in health education, because the subject was not singled out for separate provision (Whitehead, 1989; Tones, 1988). Generally, however, there was a good deal of support from teachers and professional bodies for the new developments. Moreover, it looked as if health education might consequently have a strengthened position in the new curriculum framework. This was partly due to the Act requiring schools to provide a *balanced* and *broadly based* curriculum, which not only raised educational standards, but also promoted the spiritual, moral, cultural, mental and physical development of children and prepared them for the opportunities, responsibilities and experiences of adult life (Assistant Masters and Mistresses Association (AMMA), 1989). In addition, and for the first time, health education had a small but nonetheless compulsory presence in the statutory orders for the science core subject, and schools were offered guidance on how to formulate health education policies and develop a coherent health education programme (National Curriculum Council, 1990).

However, as the full impact of the curriculum changes became clear, support for the innovation by teachers and health educationalists dwindled. Early signs indicated that some teachers were buckling under the strain of implementing the changes (Coghlan, 1989). This situation did not improve. Slater (1991) points to schools reeling from the demands of implementing the curriculum provision, of doing what Partington (1990) describes as too much, too quickly. Gillard (1992) blames the situation on the absurdity of attainment targets and statements at ten levels, constantly changing, presenting teachers with an enormous task of curriculum mapping and planning. Perhaps more significantly, Gillard (*op. cit.*) claimed that the national curriculum has pushed teachers towards a more subject orientated curriculum. It is this unfortunate emphasis on the appropriacy of subjects which has undoubtedly led to what some see as the marginalisation of health education. Mackenzie (1990) believes that core and foundation subjects are perceived as having priority because they are statutory and have been given a structure in the form of programmes of study. Teachers regard these programmes of study as their first concern because they lead to a period of testing and close reporting at the end of each key stage. The statutory attainment tests linked to some of the NC subjects have proved to be extremely time consuming, further marginalising the non-statutory areas. A further criticism of the national assessment is that it encourages staff to adopt more formal classroom approaches, as opposed to the informal, pupil-centred, teaching styles which have become associated with the delivery of health education (Troyna and Carrington, 1990; Denman, 1994).

It is commonly felt, therefore, that health education, as a cross curricular theme, has not been accorded the same status as core and foundation subjects with their statutory orders and assessment. As a consequence, health education has no authentic or credible position in the curriculum. Furthermore, Mackenzie (1990), claims that the NC cross-curricular threads are too difficult to weave into an already voluminous subject fabric. This view is shared by Ritchie (1990) who points to the *Language across the Curriculum* initiative recommended by the Bullock Report (Department for Education and Science, 1975). It is Richie's opinion that it is the failure of this and other similar initiatives that have largely discredited the idea of coordinating anything across the subject curriculum. It is important to point out, however, that this view is not shared by all. For example, Code (1990), makes a salient point when she describes health education as a subject which has always lent itself to being incorporated into other disciplines, and, in a similar way to Wragg (1990), illustrates her point by working through the science attainment targets. For the most part, however, the dominant view appears to be that the national curriculum has constrained the position of health education. O'Conner (1991) points to one significant feature of this marginalisation, the concentration of resources on the delivery of the statutory areas, including resources for in-service training. Research funded by the HEA and undertaken by the National Foundation for Educational Research (NFER) found that money for INSET courses was more likely to be available for National Curriculum foundation subjects than for health education (Health Education Authority, 1993).

A further implication of the Act is the diminished powers of teachers in terms of curriculum planning, and the increased involvement of the government and lay people in areas which were traditionally the domain of professionals. This change in power and control has resulted in an educational climate which some see as non-conducive to the enhancement of school-based health education (Denman 1994).

A key example of the diminishing powers of teachers was in evidence before the ERA. Section 46 of the 1986 Education Act gave non-education professionals, the governing bodies, choices about what should and could be taught in sex-education classes, other than the science statutory orders, and the right of veto in individual schools

(Department for Education and Science, 1986). This empowering of lay people in respect of curriculum matters has continued more recently. Section 6 of the 1993 Education Act allows parents to request withdrawal of their children wholly or partly from any lesson where sex education is taught, with the exception of national curriculum science (Morris *et al.*, 1993). As with the 1986 Act, governors were charged with overseeing policy and keeping the parents informed (Kingman, 1994). In addition to the national curriculum reforms, therefore, there has been considerable criticism of government legislation in relation to the sexual health elements of health education. This criticism has come from both educational and other professional groups (see, for example, British Medical Association, 1994; Association of School Health Education Coordinators News, 1994).

Not before time, the government has finally recognised that the implementation of the national curriculum has created considerable problems for schools, and under the leadership of Sir Ron Dearing, Chair of the School Curriculum and Assessment Authority, modifications are to be made. The most important change, as far as the future of health education is concerned, is the proposed reduction of the statutory core orders. This will allow a margin of time at each key stage, estimated as being between 15–25 per cent of total teaching time, for optional studies which can be covered at the discretion of the school. Health education was cited as one subject that could usefully be covered during the additional time released in this slimmed down curriculum (Dearing, 1994). The new statutory orders are not due to come into effect until September 1995, so any discussion of the impact these might have on health education is speculative at the time of writing. However, Brown (1994) has undertaken an analysis of the draft proposals and he believes that the slimming down of the national curriculum will result in a considerable reduction in the opportunities for health education as part of the statutory programmes of study. Whilst there may be more time for health education over and above the programmes of study, the new draft proposals suggest that there may be less scope for a cross-curricular approach. If this is indeed the case, it is crucial that teachers and other professionals with an interest in the future of health education in schools make a strong and effective case to headteachers, parents and governors for a separate provision for the subject in the margin of time within the modified national curriculum framework.

Changes in educational funding and their impact on health education

In addition to the National Curriculum, the ERA contained substantial policy shifts in relation to educational funding. The moves to both local management of schools (LMS) and to grant maintained status (GMS) have implications for the provision of health education. It is easy to discern why this might be the case. The Act fundamentally challenges the role and function of the local education authorities (LEAs), delegating many of their powers to school governing bodies and putting central services at risk (Bash and Coulby, 1989). GMS schools now buy in advisory services, for example, and both GMS and LMS schools have control over their staffing and in-service budgets.

Given the vulnerability of health education as a non-foundation subject, research indicates that it is being marginalised in the setting of priorities in relation to staffing, in-service and advisory needs (Jamison, 1993). These changes in funding arrangements will clearly have an impact on the current and future delivery of the subject.

The demise of LEA health education advisors

Another outcome of the change in LEA functions as a result of the ERA, was evidenced in the results of a recent national research study. The findings suggest that health education advisors frequently have to generate income in order to justify their positions (Scriven, 1994). The reason for this situation appears to be not only the changes in funding as a result of the ERA, but also the withdrawal of the government Grant for Education Support and Training (GEST) 12A/B. This specific funding was originally given to combat the misuse of drugs. However, the programme evolved into a preventive health initiative designed to help young people develop the skills necessary for healthy living and making healthy choices. The grant contributed substantial sums of money, £6.5 million pounds per annum, to provide skilled support for the development of schools' health education policies and programmes. This support was provided through the local education authorities by specially appointed health education coordinators. These coordinators worked closely with schools and, in many cases, also worked at the professional interface, establishing collaborative partnerships between schools, LEAs and other agencies. After seven years of GEST funding, considerable initiatives, the forerunners of *Healthy Alliances*, were in place. It is hardly surprising therefore, that when the Government decided to terminate the grant in March 1993, it was considered an outrage by all those with a vested interest in school-based health education (Lawrence, 1994; Harvey, 1993). The direct outcome of this government withdrawal of funding is a dramatic reduction in advisory support for health education (*The Times Educational Supplement*, 1993). Given the point already made concerning the marginalisation of health education as a result of changes in funding embedded in the ERA, this lack of freely provided advisory support obviously adds to the problems surrounding the continued provision and development of health education in schools. The funding changes have also come at an inopportune time, with the Department of Health calling for professionals from a range of settings to form 'healthy alliances' to address national targets set for health (Department of Health, 1992). Some of these targets are highly relevant to young people and could be usefully addressed through properly funded and coordinated health education programmes. Indeed, the then Secretary of State for Health declared schools a key setting and, in the foreword to *The Health of the Nation* document, pronounced that education was fundamental to encouraging young people to lead healthier lives. So what is the potential for healthy alliances between education and other professional groups? Unfortunately, there is clear evidence from a national audit undertaken in 1994 that although one professional group, health promotion specialists, are highly enthusiastic about working with schools and LEAs on a collaborative basis, the changes to the funding of education as a result of the ERA is making these partnerships more difficult to initiate and manage (Scriven, 1994).

Changes to the initial training of teachers

Another area of government policy which will undoubtedly influence the future delivery and development of health education in schools is the reforms to initial teacher training (ITT) (Department for Education, 1993a). Two elements in particular have direct implications. The first is the move to more school-based training, and the second is the accreditation criteria for ITT courses formulated by the Council for Accreditation of Teacher Education (CATE). The location of a significant element of training in schools will obviously disadvantage training in health education if the subject is marginalised on the curriculum. Students are unlikely to observe or be asked to be involved with health education teaching if the subject is not being taught.

Moreover, just as the National Curriculum has marginalised health education in schools, the criteria for accrediting ITT courses is marginalising the subject in the teacher training curriculum. As a subject, it is not allocated student numbers by the Government, and, since the advent of the national curriculum, both primary and secondary training courses have been measured against CATE criteria which reflect the national curriculum core and foundation subjects. The outcome of this is that students registered on a degree or postgraduate award leading to qualified teacher status are unable to choose health studies as a major in their degree programme. This is also reflected in the lack of provision for health education in the professional training elements of these courses. The exact national picture, however, is not clear. The last major survey of health education in teacher education courses took place over ten years ago. At that time, the survey indicated that there was 'a great chasm in teacher education regarding the place of health education' (Williams and Roberts, 1985, p. 46). This is a major problem, particularly as 80 per cent of students who took part in the survey said they would welcome the opportunity of teaching health education. This also explains the finding that over half of the sample group of students described their knowledge for teaching the subject as being only adequate or requiring help. It is interesting to note that 86 per cent of students in this survey thought that health education should be part of the curriculum in initial teacher training; indeed, the majority of teachers and students involved in the research said that there should be a core health education course for all students. The newly established Teacher Training Agency does not appear to have taken account of these findings when establishing current guidelines for initial teacher education programmes (Department for Education, 1993b).

There is an obvious need to update research into the extent and nature of the provision of health education in initial teacher education programmes, and an urgent requirement to establish an effective system for monitoring the impact of the Education Reform Act on the delivery of health education in schools. Recent studies, such as the HEA commissioned survey of schools' health education policies cited earlier in the chapter, indicate that all is not well. Nevertheless, the NFER project team who undertook the survey found some rays of hope. They encountered, for example, a good deal of commitment from teachers, and, where they have been appointed, school-based health education coordinators. External support has also been in evidence from school nurses, health promotion units and the LEA advisory staff still in post (for further details on school nurses, see Chapter 13). It would appear, therefore, that there is a sense of determination amongst teachers to maintain the standard of health education in schools. New initiatives such as the health promoting schools award discussed in the next chapter will undoubtedly sustain the subject through what must be regarded by all the professionals involved in its development and delivery, as a difficult period. It is hoped that the modifications made to the national curriculum will result in a more secure position for the subject at all key stages, and that the proliferation of the healthy schools awards will result in the establishment of new priorities and alliances, including a move towards more holistic approaches.

In conclusion, it is apparent that health education will continue to feature on the curriculum of schools in one form or another. It is a tragedy, however, that at a time of radical policy changes and the resultant impact on educational provision, health education has not secured a more dominant and appropriate position. Those professionals who have worked hard to establish the subject during the 1970s and 1980s will have to work with even more determination to convince education managers and policy makers of the need for a more prominent curriculum role for the subject during the latter part of the 1990s and beyond.

References

Association of School Health Education Coordinators News (1994), no. 1, January.

Assistant Masters and Mistresses Association (1989). *The National Curriculum. 'The Education Reform Act' in Focus: Guidelines for Teachers*. January. London: AMMA.

Bash, L. & Coulby, D. (1989). *The Education Reform Act: Competition and Control*. London: Cassell.

British Medical Association (1994). Press Statement. *BMA Expresses Concern that the New Education Act may Undermine Health of the Nation*. 25 February.

Brown, T. (1994). Taking the PSHE out of the national curriculum. *Health Education*, November, no. 5.

Button, L. (1984). *Developmental Group Work with Adolescents*. London: Hodder & Stoughton.

Code, T. (1990). Mapping health education topics in the NC. *Education and Health* (Nov/Dec), *8*, 71.

Coghlan, A. (1989). A bumpy path to the national curriculum. *New Scientist*, (9 December), *124*(1692), 23–24.

Dearing, R. cited in *News Focus, Health Education* (January 1994), no. 9.

Denman, S. (1994). Do schools provide an opportunity for meeting the health of the nation targets? *Journal of Public Health Medicine*, *16*(2), 219–224.

Department for Education & Science (1975) *A Language for Life*. London: HMSO.

Department for Education & Science (1986). *Health Education from 5–16: Curriculum Matters 6*. London: HMSO.

Department of Health (1992). *The Health of the Nation: A Strategy for Health in England*. London: HMSO.

Department for Education & Science (1987). *Education Reform Act*. London: HMSO.

Department for Education (1993a) The Government's Proposals for the Reforms of Initial Teacher Training. London: DFE.

Department for Education (1994b) Circular number 14/93, The Initial Training of Primary School Teachers: New Criteria for Courses. London: DFE.

Downie, R. S., Fyfe, C. & Tannahill, A. (1990). *Health Promotion: Models and Values*. Oxford: Oxford University Press.

Emmett, V. E. (1994). The future of health education. *Health Education*, May, no. 3.

Gillard, D. (1992). Educational philosophy: does it exist in the 1990's? *Forum* (Autumn), *34*(4).

Harvey, J. (1993). Health and education: partners no longer? *Public Health Alliance News*, Nov–Dec.

Health Education Authority (1993). *A Survey of Health Education Policies in Schools*. London: HEA.

Hopson, B. & Scally, M. (1981). *Lifeskills Teaching*. London: McGraw-Hill.

Jamison, J. (1993). Health education in schools: a survey of policy and implementation. *Health Education Journal* (Summer), *52*(2).

Kingman, S. (1994). The new law on sex education. *Health Education*, September, no. 4.

Lawrence, N. (1994). *ASHEC News* (January), no. 1.

Lewis, D. F. (1993). Oh for those halcyon days! A review of the development of school health education over 50 years. *Health Education Journal* (Autumn), *52*(3).

Mackenzie, C. (1990). Cross curriculum dissentions. *Education* (2 November), *176*(18).

MORI (1989). *Health Education in Schools*. Report to the Health Education Research Department, Public Health Division. London: Mori.

Morris, R., Reid, E. & Fowler, J. (1993). *Education Act '93: A Critical Guide*. London: AMMA.

Naidoo, J. & Wills, J. (1994). *Health Promotion: Foundations for Practice*. London: Bailliere Tindall.

National Curriculum Council (1990). *Curriculum Guidance 5: Health Education*. London: NCC.

O'Conner, L. (1991). Healthy nation: feeling the squeeze. *Education and Health*, *9*(2).

Partington, J. (1990). Week by week. *Education* (6 July), *176*.

Ritchie, H. (1990). Out of the frying pan, into the teapot. *Education* (23 November), *176*.

Scriven, A. (1994). Results of a national audit of healthy alliances between NHS specialist health promotion units and schools/LEAs. Unpublished research report. Bath College of Higher Education.

Scriven, A. (1995). Not a good year for health education. *Health Education* (January), no. 1.

Slater, D. (1991). Prospecting fools gold: auditing the curriculum. *Forum* (Spring), *33*(2).

The Times Educational Supplement (1993), January 8, as reported in J. Jamison (1993), *op. cit.*

Tones, K. (1988). The role of the school in health promotion: the primacy of personal and social education. in *Westminster Studies in Education*, *11*.

Tones, K. & Tilford, S. (1990). *Health Education: Effectiveness and Efficiency*. London: Chapman & Hall.

Troyna, B. & Carrington, B. (1990). *Education, Racism and Reform*. London: Routledge.

Whitehead, M. (1989). *Swimming Upstream: Trends and Prospects in Education for Health*. London: King's Fund Institute.

Williams, T. & Roberts, J. (1985). *Health Education in Schools and Teacher Education Institutions*. London: Health Education Council.

Wragg, T. (1990). You can do health education in the NC. *Education and Health* (March/April), *8*.

12 The health promoting school: from idea to action

Alan Beattie

The concept of the health promoting school concerns the school as a total environment, beyond the teaching about health matters that happens in classrooms, and the medical and nursing attention that pupils receive through school health services. An influential recent publication puts it as follows:

> The health promoting school aims at achieving healthy lifestyles for the total school population by developing supportive environments conducive to the promotion of health.
>
> It offers opportunities for, and requires commitments to, the provision of a safe and health-enhancing social and physical environment.
>
> (World Health Organisation, 1993).

The idea that the school as an institution is a suitable arena for action to promote health is not in itself new. Since around 1900, schools have been test-beds in which children (easily seen, easily examined and easily described) have been subjected to analysis and intervention in the name of wider regimes of public health (Armstrong, 1993a). For the first 50 years of this century, medical advice was a dominant influence on the architecture and management of schools. This advice led to the replacement of the previous central-hall plan by new corridor, quadrangle and finger plans, on sanitary principles. It was believed that the new form would provide better ventilation and lighting, and it continued to dominate school architecture until the late 1950s (Lowe, 1973). Alongside this, new systems were brought in for the medical inspection of children, and for the provision of physical drills and of school meals. These introduced for the first time an emphasis on the personal health and hygiene of the individual pupil (Armstrong, 1993b).

Textbooks in use for trainee teachers in the 1960s continued to deal with school premises as an aspect of hygiene and health education (for example Davies, 1962; Gamlin, 1959). But from the 1950s to the 1990s, the previous emphasis on the school environment as an influ-

ence on health, and indeed the use of the term hygiene, moved off the
agenda, as attention shifted to pupil lifestyles and the psychosocial
origins of risk-taking behaviour (as in smoking, drinking, drug use,
relationships and sexuality). The growth of interest in the past few
years in the health promoting school is an example of the re-establish-
ment of an ecological view of health that is one of the hallmarks of the
new public health and the settings-based approach (Baric, 1993;
Ashton and Seymour, 1988). It reflects a new concern to address at
one and the same time both the individual lifestyles of pupils and the
corporate life of the school as an organisation, as can be seen in the
ten aims set out by the WHO (*Table 12.1*).

It was experience in curriculum development for health education
in British schools that led to some of the earliest observations on the
need to follow through what is learned in the classroom, as a matter

Table 12.1   *Aims of the European network of health promoting schools*

---

1 Provide a health promoting environment for working and learning
   through its buildings, play areas, catering facilities, safety measures, etc.

2 Promote individual, family and community responsibility for health.

3 Encourage healthy lifestyles and present a realistic and attractive
   range of health choices for schoolchildren and staff.

4 Enable all pupils to fulfil their physical, psychological and social
   potential and promote their self-esteem.

5 Set out clear aims for the promotion of health and safety for the
   whole school community (children and adults).

6 Foster good pupil–pupil and staff–pupil relationships and good
   links between the school, the home and the community.

7 Exploit the availability of community resources to support action for
   the promotion of health.

8 Plan a coherent health education curriculum with educational
   methods that actively engage pupils.

9 Equip pupils with the knowledge and skills they need both to make
   sound decisions about their personal health and to preserve and
   improve a safe and healthy physical environment.

10 Take a wide view of school health services as an educational
   resource that can help pupils become effective health care consu-
   mers.

Source: World Health Organisation, 1993

of practice throughout the whole school environment and in the everyday daily life of the school (Williams, 1985). But as with many other aspects of the new public health, European policy-making bodies have been prominent in taking forward the idea of the health promoting school The European Community Council of Ministers of Education issued a resolution encouraging authorities within member states to make arrangements to develop schools as settings for health promotion (European Commission, 1989), and the European Network of Health Promoting Schools referred to above (which currently involves over 30 European countries) is a joint research and development initiative of the WHO European Office, the Council of Europe and the Commission of the European Communities.

Table 12.2 *Criteria for a health promoting school*

1 The active promotion of the self-esteem of all pupils by demonstrating that everyone can make a contribution to the life of the school.

2 The development of good relations between staff and pupils and between pupils in the daily life of the school.

3 The clarification for staff and pupils of the social aims of the school.

4 The provision of stimulating challenges for all pupils through a wide range of activities.

5 Using every opportunity to enhance the physical environment of the school.

6 The development of good links between the school, the home and the community.

7 The development of good links between associated primary and secondary schools to plan a coherent health education curriculum.

8 The active promotion of the health and well-being of school staff.

9 The consideration of the role of staff exemplars in health-related issues.

10 The consideration of the complementary role of school meals (if provided) to the health education curriculum.

11 The employment of specialist services in the community for advice and support in health matters.

12 The development of the education potential of the school health services beyond routine screening towards active support for the health education curriculum.

Source: based on HEA, 1993

In England, the National Curriculum Council guidance on health education included a section on a *whole-school approach* which draws attention of the subtle messages that pupils receive about health from the daily life of the school, and to the other factors that may impinge on its effectiveness as a health promotion setting, such as the organisation and management structures of a school, its physical environment, and its links with the local community (National Curriculum Council, 1990). Subsequently *The Health of the Nation* endorsed the idea of setting up a pilot network of health promoting schools (Department of Health, 1992). The Health Education Authority has adopted the criteria devised by the European Network, and any participating school is expected to agree to work towards meeting these (see *Table 12.2*).

During 1995, 16 pilot schools in England, selected after a major audit study by an independent research agency National Foundation

---

Table 12.3   *Key areas for action to create a healthy school*

---

1   *Curriculum* The school should be working towards the NCC Guidance No 5. Its policies and programmes should be coordinated, comprehensive and progressive, and be reflected in the School Development Plan.

2   *Environment* The school should promote a stimulating, clean and safe environment.

3   *Policy* Policies should reflect the school as a health-promoting environment which is part of the wider community.

4   *Hygiene* The school should promote hygienic practices.

5   *Safety* The school should promote a safe environment; this includes physical, personal and psychological safety.

6   *Exercise and activity* The school should offer a wide range of physical activities which are accessible to all and in which working towards an active lifestyle becomes an important cultural practice within the school.

7   *Food* Pupils should be educated and encouraged to make healthy food choices.

8   *Smoking* The school should be working towards a smoke-free environment.

9   *Management* There should be a holistic approach to the management of health-promoting issues in the school.

Source: Mancunian Community Health NHS Trust Health Promotion Service and Manchester City Council Inspection and Advisory Service (1994)

for Educational Research (NFER), have begun to implement three-year development plans, with support and monitoring from the HEA. Some local authorities have devised their own schemes for encouraging work on healthy school initiatives, as in the Manchester example summarised in *Table 12.3*.

A shortage of serious action

From the foregoing, it is clear that the idea of the health promoting school is by now popular among planners at international, national and regional levels. But the evidence on implementation at school level is rather discouraging. A survey carried out in 1992 by NFER of a representative sample of primary and secondary schools in England, found that there was widespread support for the idea of health education as an important function of schools, and that some recognised the value of a health promoting school (Jamison, 1993). But it found also that a large number of schools are still in the process of developing a written policy document, and it identified widespread concern about the shortage of suitable trained staff, and the shortage of time and money to secure appropriate training, especially faced with a perceived marginalisation of health education by the statutory requirements of National Curriculum subjects (see further discussion of this in Chapter 11). A systematic series of studies in Wales has likewise highlighted the large gap between the theory and the practice of the health promoting school (Nutbeam *et al.*, 1987; Nutbeam, 1992; Smith *et al.*, 1992; Smith *et al.*, 1994). Despite widespread commitment to the value of health promotion activity, whole school policies as regards smoking had been developed in only a minority of schools. Policies for healthy eating had been developed in even fewer schools; while genuinely active involvement of parents in school health promotion policies was rare. The Welsh studies also found that opportunities for inservice training were seen as inadequate for the take up of good practice in connection with the health promoting school. This mixed response on the part of schools is illustrated in comments from two senior staff that were interviewed in the summer of 1991 as part of a feasibility study for the HEA on setting up a Healthy Schools support scheme (Beattie, 1991):

> ... the school as a health promoting environment is a really good idea. It's a basis for a holistic approach and helps you attack double standards across the whole school community. Staff would welcome it too.
>
> (A Deputy Head in a high school in Wigan)

...a health promoting school scheme is a good idea. The problem will be to find time to do it. We scarcely touch health as an aspect of the whole school environment.

(A health education coordinator in a high school in London)

It seems clear that the future development of health promoting schools will depend in large part on the prospects for the funding of in-service training for teachers. If there is any way forward that offers promise, perhaps it lies in seeking to develop closer alliances between schools and the health services, especially the purchasing authorities who are now charged with looking after the health of their local populations. This case has recently been argued by Turner (1994):

If primary schools are to become more health promoting in both their practice and ethos, then it is important that they actively seek information about, and gain access to and support from an appropriate range of District Health Authority (DHA) services. DHAs must also be pro-active in making links with the primary schools within their boundaries, if they are serious about improving both the present and future health status of the children they serve.

Turner goes on to observe that in the context of such collaborative arrangements, it will also be important to address differences in style and practice in health promotion, and the different values and beliefs that underlie these, which (as he points out) are currently a focus of lively theoretical debate in the health promotion world. Indeed, as Ewles and Simnett (1992, p. 20) indicate, health promotion is an umbrella term for a wide range of activities, and there is no single or widely adopted consensus on what may be included under this term. However, in the past few years it has become increasingly common among health promotion planners and practitioners to make use of one or more published frameworks for reviewing the range of possible health promotion approaches and for designing a specific project or programme. In the remainder of this chapter, I want to examine some of the *tools of thought* that can help to make a reality of the health promoting school.

Frameworks for developing 'health school' plans

The various conceptual frameworks (or models) for health promotion planning that have come into use provide tools for dealing with the *dilemmas of choice* that arise in deciding on the form that an initiative should take. They offer a way of reflecting on and clarifying the different sorts of aims, purposes, targets, procedures (and underlying values) that may need to be taken into account in a particular situation; and they can prompt those involved in a planning process to work out for themselves which aims, activities and values they can agree to proceed with (Ewles and Simnett 1992, pp. 35–38). Another recent textbook for health promotion practitioners observes that:

> Using a model can be helpful because it encourages you to think theoretically, and come up with new strategies and ways of working. It can also help you to prioritize and locate more or less desirable types of interventions.

> (Naidoo and Wills, 1994, p. 93)

In what follows, four different frameworks will be set out that offer promise in the present context. As will be seen, each of them can serve to highlight some particular dilemmas and issues in putting together a development plan for a health promoting school.

The Tannahill model

This framework identifies three distinct (but overlapping) elements that make up the field of contemporary health promotion activity. It was devised by a specialist (Tannahill, 1985) in public health medicine working in the NHS context, and was adopted by what was

Table 12.4 *The Tannahill framework applied to developing the health promoting school*

Disease prevention	Health education	Health protection
Clinical activity that prevents (or reduces risk of) illness, injury, disability, handicap	Communications that influence knowledge, beliefs and behaviour that affect health	Codes of administrative practice, and legal or fiscal control that promote health
For example: • medical screening • child immunization • fitness testing	For example: • health education • personal-social education • social and lifeskills – curriculum and resources	For example: • designated no-smoking areas • stress management policies • additives-free catering

Source: modified from Downie *et al.*, 1990; Evans and Lee, 1990; Joyce and Binstead, 1990; Turner, 1994

probably the first national project to develop guidelines for working towards the health promoting school (Evans and Lee, 1990; Joyce and Binstead, 1990). These authors use the model as a central part of a process for setting up a health promoting institution. Turner (1994) has also made brief reference to the same model in the context of purchasing practical health promotion for the primary school. *Table 12.4* sets out a summary of the key elements of the Tannahill framework and of some of the forms of action which can be encompassed within each of the headings within the framework.

It may be noted that this framework pulls together health promotion through the curriculum and through the school health service (as described later in Chapter 13), and adds to these the regulatory level that appears under the health protection heading. The origins of this model and its current applications lie clearly within a medical context, and it may be that it is of most use in supporting dialogue between schools and health service colleagues.

The Ryder and Campbell model

This framework was devised by two educationalists involved in the development of good practice in health education and pastoral care in schools (Ryder and Campbell, 1988). They offer a scheme for examin-

Table 12.5   *The Ryder and Campbell 'PERM' framework for developing PSHE*

Pastoral/ individual	Educational/ rational	Radical/political	Medical/ traditional
Fosters self-esteem and self-empowerment	Provides access to knowledge, understanding and reasoning	Encourages group action to undertake critical analysis and problem-solving	Promotes compliance with objective expert advice
via, for example: • roleplay • simulations trust exercises	via, for example: • checklists • debates • investigations	via, for example: • local community surveys • monitoring of mass media	via, for example: • posters • lectures • films • worksheets • leaflets

Source: modified from Ryder and Campbell 1988, chapter 3

ing the advantages and disadvantages of four different approaches to the personal-social-health education (PSHE) curriculum, in terms of a scheme (so-called PERM) which is based on a range of earlier work by others in this area). These authors also offer suggestions for embedding PSHE within a process of organisational development for 'the healthy school'; and they outline an agenda for taking forward work on the 'whole school climate' and the 'organisational health' of the school as an institution. *Table 12.5* sets out a summary of some key elements in the PERM scheme and the aims and forms of action that it encompasses:

Ryder and Campbell show how the PERM scheme can be used as what they call a ready reckoner to assess and compare a variety of teaching methods and exercises, or curriculum resource packs, as a means of clarifying aims and achievements and also of checking out what may be considered an ideal balance of different approaches. Tantalisingly, they do not fully develop the links between PERM-analysis and the processes of working towards the healthy school as a whole, but they do offer a *four-tier model* which they suggest can connect desired PSHE outcomes for staff and students with the values of healthy organisational life. This is summarised in *Table 12.6*.

Ryder and Campbell's work offers some challenging ideas for prompting critical and creative work on developing the health promoting school; their argument is that organisational development (towards healthier schools) depends crucially on the kinds of values that are central to PSHE itself. It's perhaps relevant to point out that their discussion is in language that springs very clearly from the world of educationalists, and that it may therefore find its greatest

Table 12.6 *Ryder and Campbell's model of 'healthy organisational life' in schools*

Individual outcomes	Peer group outcomes	Institutional outcomes	Community outcomes
Self-confidence Independence in learning Problem-solving	Collaboration and sharing Communication and feedback Challenging stereotypes	Healthier climate Goals more overt, less covert Visible, open and participative decisions	Community involvement Sociopolitical engagement 'Healthier' society

Source: modified from Ryder and Campbell, 1988, chapter 7

utility in helping staff in schools to explore and identify their own common ground, perhaps even before joint work with NHS colleagues.

The Ewles and Simnett model

This framework identifies five separate frameworks that come under the umbrella of health promotion work. It was devised by two specialist health promotion practitioners (Ewles and Simnett, 1992, p. 37), and is to be found in wide use (see, for example, Naidoo and Wills, 1994, p. 92), most commonly applied to the analysis and planning of action on specific health topics, such as smoking cessation or healthy eating. However, one recent publication has noticed the potential of

Table 12.7   *The Ewles and Simnett framework and the school as a healthy workplace*

Approach	Aim	Activity
Medical	Identify those at risk	Provide screening; provide immunization
Behaviour change	Encourage individual responsibility	Require compliance with policies (for example, safety; no smoking)
Educational	Increase knowledge and skills	Health education programmes for pupils; health education training courses for staff
Empowerment	Work with clients on their own agendas	Support staff self-help groups (for example, stop smoking; weight control); pastoral/PSHE programmes for pupils
Social change	Modify the physical and social environment	Set up safety policies (in light of legal directives, for example EC); develop workplace smoking policy

Source: modified from Ewles and Simnett, 1992, p. 37; Naidoo and Wills, 1994, p. 92; Molloy, 1995, p. 150

this model for exploring the settings-based approach to health promotion, namely the case of the workplace (Molloy, 1995, p. 150). Set out in *Table 12.7* is a summary of the key features of the Ewles and Simnett framework as it might be applied in the context of the school as a health promoting workplace.

One strength of the Ewles and Simnett model is that it is descriptive of what health promoters commonly do; and this tabulation can help to underline the idea that the school is a workplace like any other. As such, it presents an opportunity to develop a health promotion strategy which attends to the whole school, as an environment for employees as well as for pupils. It might be of particular value in whole school staff development sessions, or in discussions within the governing body.

The Beattie model

This model offers a structural analysis of the repertoire of health promotion, identifying two distinct dimensions along which strategies may differ, and around which there is often considerable dispute (Beattie, 1991b). In *Figure 12.1*, the vertical refers to the mode of intervention which ranges along a spectrum from authoritative (top-down, expert-directed) to negotiated (bottom-up, reflecting the agreed agendas of individual or group clients). The horizontal dimension refers to the focus of intervention, which similarly ranges along a spectrum of work with an individual (one to one), to work with groups, with communities, and with whole corporate bodies. The resulting matrix is a way of mapping the strategic choices that face

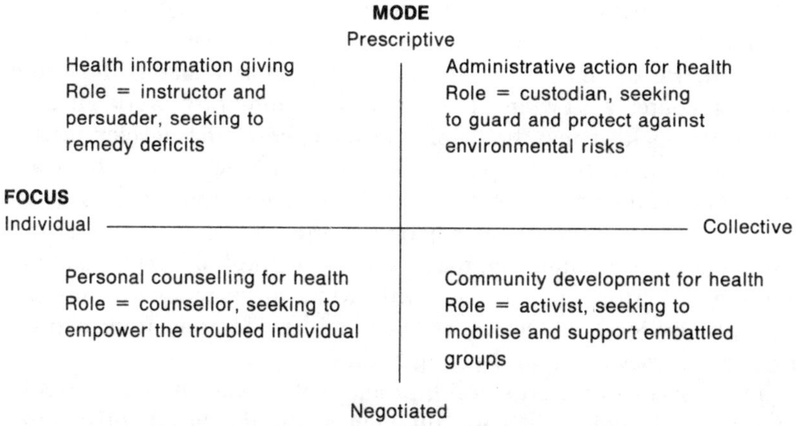

MODE
Prescriptive

Health information giving	Administrative action for health
Role = instructor and	Role = custodian, seeking
persuader, seeking to	to guard and protect against
remedy deficits	environmental risks

FOCUS
Individual ——————————————————————————— Collective

Personal counselling for health	Community development for health
Role = counsellor, seeking to	Role = activist, seeking to
empower the troubled individual	mobilise and support embattled
	groups

Negotiated

Figure 12.1   *Beattie's matrix of health promotion strategies*

those involved in health promotion planning and provision, in terms of four distinct clusters of activity. It can be useful both in charting and selecting the particular mix of approaches that may make up any specific programme or project, and also in exploring and reviewing the ethical and political tensions within an intervention in terms of the balance of social values that it encompasses (Beattie, 1993). The model has been applied to schools (Beattie, 1984), where it helps to clarify the tensions that arise between health promotion through (say) the science curriculum, through pastoral care and casework with individual pupils, through the encouragement of environmental awareness and action, and through the fostering of community participation and local action.

However, the case of development planning for health promoting schools, as an extremely interesting and valuable line of work that has emerged in the past few years, which has adapted and extended the Beattie model as a basis for applying the settings-based approach to health promotion in Colleges of Further Education (O'Donnell and Gray, 1993). This consultancy project (funded by the Health Education Authority) has worked with a large sample of Colleges around England, and has devised a series of planning grids which are used to depict and summarise the range of options open to Colleges in their efforts to develop policies at a corporate level for handling, for example, smoking cessation and stress management across the whole College. The work of O'Donnell and Gray has identified a useful additional dimension, which spells out four different levels in the corporate life and policy of a College at which the matrix can be applied. *Table 12.8* sets out a version of a planning grid, which has been modified in turn (after O'Donnell and Gray) in the light of further work on this approach carried out in a current project which is allying the settings-based approach to the development of a health promoting campus in a higher education institution (Beattie, 1995).

In addition to its use in health promotion in school and college settings, the Beattie matrix has also been adopted and adapted for use in nursing contexts (Twinn, 1991) and in community work (Beattie, 1986). As such, it may be helpful in dialogue in the development of healthy alliances across agency boundaries, between the school and the NHS, and/or between the school and adult education or youth and community services. Furthermore, the emphasis in this framework on the corporate approach can be helpful in joint planning, audit and performance review with wider managerial systems; for example, by local inspectors, assessors and moderators from national project schemes and award-giving bodies.

The movement towards health promoting schools offers the promise of refreshing and revitalising thinking about the health of children and young people, and could have important knock-on effects for

Table 12.8 *The Beattie matrix as a planning grid for the health promoting school*

Health information & advice-giving to redirect the behaviour of individuals	Talks/films/ seminars on the risks of smoking, HIV/ AIDS, etc.	Exhibitions/ events on current health topics	Set aside space and resources for health promotion activities	Develop policies on individual risks, e.g. whole school smoking policies
Personal counselling for health to support life-review & self-empowered change	Discussions & role play on peer pressures and social skills in health, e.g. drugs, alcohol, smoking	Opportunities and support for self-review and self-help	Facilities for self-help & group work	Policies to support staff who need to adapt to new rules and codes, e.g. smoking
Administrative action for health to reform administrative/ regulatory systems	Assignments & projects which explore & assess the health profile of the school	Forums for review and participation in decision-making about 'healthy school' issues	Labelling, signposting, and way finding to support a 'healthy school' ethos	Fully worked out school policies and rules re health, agreed with governors & parents
Community development for health to identify common ground & facilitate joint action	Courses for parent education; allied adult and community education courses	Meetings, forums, fairs, street events to open up debate & decision-making about the 'healthy school'	Provide for dual and multiple use of space and resources: 'Healthy school = open school'?	Fully worked out policies and guidelines re outreach, placements, liaison, etc.

Source: modified after Beattie, 1984, 1991b, 1995; O'Donnell and Gray, 1993

school staff, for families and for local communities. The support schemes that are being put into place may be a crucial way of making a reality of the ideal of *Health for All*. But to bring this to pass, those involved in the action must be fully aware of the current debate about different ways of undertaking health promotion, and about the different value positions that are at stake in this line of work. As one health promotion practitioner, active and committed in the schools context, put it (Beattie, 1991a):

Focusing on the school as a health promoting environment should be the abiding principle. An award scheme would be very good in encouraging this – as long as it didn't fall into the trap of favouring a medical model...

References

Armstrong, D. (1993a). Public health spaces and the fabrication of identity. *Sociology*, *27*, 3, 393–410.

Armstrong, D (1993b). From clinical gaze to regime of total health. In A. Beattie, L. Jones, M. Gott, & M. Sidell (eds), *Health and Wellbeing: A Reader*. London: Macmillan.

Ashton, J., & Seymour, H. (1988). *The New Public Health*. Buckingham: Open University Press.

Baric, L. (1993). The settings approach: implications for policy and strategy. *Journal of the Institute of Health Education*, *30*(1), 17–24.

Beattie, A. (1984). Health education and the science teacher: invitation to a debate. *Education and Health* (January), 9–15.

Beattie, A. (1986). Community development for health: from practice to theory? *Radical Health Promotion*, *4*, 11–16.

Beattie, A. (1991a). *Supporting School Health Education in the Context of the National Curriculum*. Research Report for the Young People's Programme. London: HEA.

Beattie, A. (1991b). Knowledge and control in health promotion: a test-case for social theory and social policy. In J. Gabe, M. Calnan & M. Bury (eds), *Sociology of the Health Service*. London: Routledge.

Beattie, A. (1993). The changing boundaries of health. In A. Beattie, M. Gott, L. Jones, & M. Sidell (eds), *Health and Wellbeing: A Book of Readings*. London: Macmillan.

Beattie, A. (1995). The health promoting campus: a case study in project-based learning and competency profiling. In A. Edwards and P. Knight (eds), *Degrees of Competence: The Assessment of Competence in Higher Education*. Chapter 9. London: Kogan Page.

Davies, M. B. (1962). *Hygiene and Health Education for Training Colleges*, 9th ed. London: Longmans.

Department of Health (1992). *The Health of the Nation*. London: HMSO.

Downie, R. S., Fyfe, C. & Tannahill, A. (1990). *Health Promotion Models and Values*. Oxford: Oxford Medical.

European Commission (1989). Resolution of Council of Ministers of Education, meeting within Council 23. November, 1988, concerning health education in schools. *European Commission Official Journal* 89/c/3/01.

Evans, V. & Lee, J. (1990). *Health Promoting Schools: A Training Manual*. Salford: The Advisory Council on Alcohol and Drug Education.

Ewles, L. & Simnett, I. (1992). *Promoting Health: A Practical Guide*. London: Scutari Press.

Gamlin, R. (1959). *Modern School Hygiene*, 19th edn. Welwyn: Nisbet.

Health Education Authority (1993). *The Concept of the Health Promoting School: The European Network of Health Promoting Schools – How Your School can be Involved*. London: HEA.

Hovey, A. (1993). *Creating a Smoke Free School*. Cardiff: Health Promotion Authority for Wales.

Jamison, J. (1993). Health Education in schools. A survey of policy and implementation. *Health Education Journal, 52*, 2, 59–62.

Joyce, R. & Binstead, M. (1990). *Health Promoting Schools: A Process Document*. Cambridge: Cambridge Health Promotion Service.

Lowe, R. A. (1973). *The medical profession and school design in England, 1902–1914. Pedagogica Historica 13*, 2, 425–444.

Mancunian Community Health NHS Trust Health Promotion Service and Manchester City Council Inspection and Advisory Service (1994). *Manchester Healthy School Award Scheme: Information Planner*. Manchester: Withington Hospital.

Molloy, J. (1995). Health promotion in the workplace. In M. Bamford (ed.), *Work and Health*. Chapter 6. London: Chapman & Hall.

Naidoo, J. & Wills, J. (1994). *Health Promotion: Foundations for Practice*. London: Bailliere Tindall.

National Curriculum Council (1990). *Curriculum Guidance 5: Health Education*. York: NCC.

Nutbeam, D., Clarkson, J., Phillips, K., Everett, V., Hill, A. & Catford, J. (1987). The health promoting school: organisation and policy development in Welsh secondary schools. *Health Education Journal, 46*, 3, 109–15.

Nutbeam, D. (1992). The health promoting school: closing the gap between theory and practice. *Health Promotion International, 7*, 3, 151–153.

O'Donnell, T. & Gray, G. (1993). *The Health Promoting College*. London: HEA.

Rawson, D. (1992). The growth of health promotion theory. In R. Bunton & G. Macdonald (eds), *Health Promotion: Disciplines and Diversity*. London: Routledge.

Ryder, J. & Campbell, L. (1988). *Balancing Acts in Personal Social and Health Education*. London: Routledge.

Scottish Health Education Group (1990). *Promoting Good Health: Proposals for Action in Schools*. Edinburgh: Scottish Health Education Group.

Smith, C., Roberts, C., Nutbeam, D. & Macdonald, G. (1992). The health promoting school: progress and future challenges in Welsh secondary schools. *Health Promotion International, 7*, 171–179.

Smith, C., Frankland, J., Playle, R. & Moore, L. (1994). A survey of health promotion in Welsh primary schools 1993. *Health Education Journal, 53*, 237–248.

Tannahill, A. (1985). What is health promotion? *Health Education Journal, 44*, 167–168.

Turner, R. (1994). Purchasing practical health promotion for the primary school: a DHA perspective. In R. Morton & J. Lloyd (eds), *The Health Promoting Primary School*. Chapter 2. London: Fulton.

Twinn, S. F. (1991). Conflicting paradigms of health visiting: a continuing debate for professional practice. *Journal of Advanced Nursing, 16*, 966–973.

World Health Organisation (1993). *The European Network of Health Promoting Schools*. Copenhagen: WHO (Euro).

Williams, T. (1985). Health education and the school/community interface. In G. Campbell (ed.), *New Directions in Health Education*. Brighton: Falmer.

Young, I. & Williams, T. (1989). *The Healthy School*. Edinburgh: SHEG.

13 *The role of the school nurse in promoting health*

Stephen Farrow

When services become invisible they run the risk of being reduced or even abandoned. During the 1980s, the school health service was such a service (Harrison and Gretton, 1986) and in many parts of the country it suffered significant cuts. These changes came about partly because people believed that the improved socioeconomic circumstances of children and families, when compared with their counterparts in the early decades of this century, did not require a service whose origins lay in poverty. They also resulted from a lack of clarity of the role of the school nurse and concern for the cost effectiveness of the school health service. The original role of the school nurse was, after all, to focus on the detection and treatment of poor hygiene, infestations and malnutrition and to provide a supporting role to school medical officers. The 1944 Education Act had extended the work of the school nurse to the secondary school; the 1981 Education Act had integrated children with learning difficulties into ordinary schools; and the national curriculum (1989) introduced the requirement to provide for health education and health promotion. In general, the post-war period had seen increased opportunities and increased activity particularly in the field of immunisation and health promotion. At the same time, however, there was a reduction in the numbers of community medical officers working in schools and an alteration in the general relationships between nurses and doctors with greater autonomy of school nurses. At the very same time that opportunities have increased for school nurses to have a greater impact on the health of children, there has been a general questioning of their role and, more particularly, the level of resources that should be allocated to children, schools, health education and health promotion.

One aspect of the developing debate has been the training and education of school nurses themselves. Before 1974, most school nurses were trained health visitors but the number holding this qualification has been steadily declining (Doggett *et al.*, 1992).

Before describing the role of school nurses in health promotion and the current constraints to and opportunities for the development of their role, a brief review of the literature will be attempted. It begins with comments on the historical context and the organisation of school nursing services, and a discussion of the nurses' role. This is followed by a brief reference to the debate over school medicals, school inspections and the screening interview. The next sections consider the general question of workload and training needs, and a series of specific issues which illustrate various expanding aspects of the current job. The final section deals with health promotion in particular, and what factors may influence its development.

Historical context and organisation

School nursing has been in transition since its inception, and the role of the school nurse as primary care coordinator, school health coordinator, case manager and epidemiologist is replacing outdated nursing functions (Igoe, 1994). Nevertheless, it is important to recall the history of school nursing and the fact that Amy Hughes and a small group of nurses had been instrumental in the founding of school and district nursing over 100 years ago (Vine, 1991).

In a contribution to the 'Whither health visiting' series in Health Visitor, Bagnall (1989) concluded that the school nursing service needed a thorough review and update. Given the stated importance of the child at the political level and the emergence of key policy documents (Primary Health Care Group, 1988; Health Visitors Association, 1988), it was time for school nurses and managers to implement some of the changes that were obviously needed.

Another perspective comes from reports of school nursing services within different districts in England. Norwich has one of the most comprehensive programmes of school nurse activities including screening at entrance, systematically throughout the child's career and health interviews. Discussions take place about future careers with special attention given to medical conditions. There is an extensive programme of health education regarding diet, exercise, smoking and other relevant subjects. Counselling, if necessary, for any health, social and personal worries is also provided as are drop-in clinics (Hawes, 1989).

Compared to Norwich, there are many districts with only a skeleton school health or school nursing service. It is also quite common to find two districts in the same region with quite different approaches to school nursing. In Bristol, in 1992, a consultation document suggested saving £250 000 from the school nurse establishments in order to buy in health promotion and to provide paramedical services for children with special needs. In contrast, in Exeter, the school nurse was placed at the heart of services for children (Jackson, 1992).

In Stockport, the school health strategy involved the development of teams consisting of a health visitor (G Grade), school nurse (C–F Grade) and health care assistant (Jackson, 1991). A slightly different approach to team working was introduced in Wandsworth. A restructuring of the schools' programme led to the introduction of team working and a greater emphasis on health promotion. The team there is essentially an F grade school nurse team leader, a D grade nurse and a clerical officer (Turner, 1994). In East Dorset the school nursing service is introducing nursery nurses alongside school nurses (Lochhead, 1994).

In the United States, both the history and the changes have been similar to those described above. In fact the challenge for school nursing is as great today as it was in 1902 when Lilian Wald first identified the need for school nurses. In Michigan, public schools have not employed school nurses for over a decade. One way round the difficulty of the public funding of school nurses has been to look to the nursing faculties who have placed student nurses within the school system. Students have carried out a variety of projects including suicide prevention, disaster response, nutrition and personnel hygiene (Czajka and George, 1991).

The list of services provided by school nurses that the National Association of State School Nurse Consultants believe should be eligible for Medicaid Funding includes: case finding; nursing care procedures; care coordination; patient/student counselling/instruction; and emergency care (National Association of State School Nurse Consultants, 1993). In the United States, there have been increasing pressures for schools to take greater responsibility for providing health care. Thurber *et al.* (1991) have described the different state mandates for health education and the role of the school nurses in health education.

Comparisons between the United Kingdom and the United States experience have been described by Thompson (1989). Her observations include salary differences, working conditions, professional preparation and professional recognition.

The role of school nurses

Surveys of the views of pupils and staff on the role of the school nurse have shown that they tended to view the nurse in a traditional way, that is, tending to the sick and injured, whereas the nurse tended to give priority to health surveillance, screening and prevention of illness together with health promotion (Staunton, 1983; Hansen, 1987; Adams, 1990). The views of parents differed in that they saw routine medicals, hygiene inspections, and regular vision and hearing tests as important (Cutting and Fahey, 1988; Fahey and

Cutting, 1988, 1989; Adams, 1990). From these findings and those from North America it could be said that parents had the most limited perception of the school nurse's role (Greenhill, 1979). Parents and teachers are often seen as authority figures, whereas the school nurse is seen as an independent health professional. Cohen (1994) gives examples of the collaboration between school nurses and teachers. A survey was conducted in Ottawa schools before the introduction of a compulsory AIDS education programme. Girls considered parents, and boys considered school nurses, to be the next most credible source of information (Dolan *et al.*, 1990).

An important aspect of the role of school nurses is the extent to which they take a leadership role within the school. With the introduction of new programmes, such as the care of the pregnant teenager and substance-abuse education, the school nurse was increasingly involved with other professionals both inside an outside the school system. The nurses' effectiveness depended greatly on their ability to lead (Adams, 1991).

Despite the widening of the role, the school nurse functions may not be that visible to schoolchildren themselves. A review of children in Bath showed that for pupils entering secondary school, the children were aware of who the school nurse was and how to contact her but were unaware of what she did (Williamson, 1992). Several authors have stressed the enormous variation in the roles of school nurses across the country and the necessary competencies to make the role successful (Parsons and Felton, 1992; Yates, 1992; While and Barriball, 1993).

The Health Visitors Association's policy document *Project Health* was launched in 1991 to coincide with the first national school nursing week. It was the intention of the professional organisation to bring school nursing out of the cupboard and onto the community nursing agenda.What was identified was a general lack of understanding amongst community nurse managers of the role of the school nurse (Bagnall, 1991). Orr (1991) emphasised the importance of developing standards for school nurses. Bays (1991) discussed the importance of effectiveness of programmes in enhancing the image of the school nurse. This raises the question of what would be useful outcome criteria. Two suggestions have been utilisation of health services and student time lost from school (Jones and Clark, 1993).

Medicals or screening interviews

Until 1959, all children on entry to school were required to have a medical inspection. After that date, many health authorities offered medical examination to parents on a voluntary basis. By 1985 it is estimated that 90 per cent of parents were receiving such an offer but by 1991 the number had probably dropped to 75 per cent. Bax and Whitmore (1991) argue that the medical examination provides unique opportunities to assess the child and to take a holistic view about the child's health. This was also supported by Elliott *et al.* They audited the school health records of 1127 Cheshire schoolchildren and noted wide variation in referral rates. There were abnormalities detected amongst 45 per cent of the children that had not previously been detected, with 21 per cent needing referral (Elliott *et al.*, 1994).

This view, however, is not universally shared. Bolton (1994) described the replacement of the conventional school medical with a new system of screening school entrants by the school nurse in the Canterbury and Thanet health district. Not only was the system satisfactory to children and parents, it increased the school nurse's job satisfaction and was said to be more cost effective. Houghton *et al.* (1992) proposed a similar system following a detailed study of 82 consecutive examinations performed by four school doctors on children aged over five. In Ealing, the health interview is the key part of the process of identifying children with health needs for medical examination, and is conducted on all primary school entrants. The new programme not only releases school nurse time for developing health promotion activities within the core curriculum it also acknowledges the important lead role of the school nurse within the school health service (Mattock, 1991).

In general, the objection to routine school medicals, including those for school leavers, concerns their cost-effectiveness, in view of the small number of new problems that are detected (Roberts, 1993).

Current workload and training needs

Many authors have described the size of the case load. In Norwich, the caseload for individual nurses ranged from 400 to 1500 pupils (Hawes, 1989). Adams (1992) reports on the workload of a particular school nurse in the school system in the United States, who covers 2500 pupils in one high school, one junior high school and three elementary schools.

Increasing activity has usually been accompanied by a large increase in clerical work, and that is equally true when there is an increase in health education and health promotion (Nelson, 1989). Hunter (1991) studied the variety of tasks by using a diary of activities during a one-week period, and concluded that routine tasks were getting in the way of others (health promotion) which might be more productive. This same point was made by Kobokovich and Bonovich (1992) in relation to adolescent pregnancy prevention activities.

Districts that have established strong school nursing programmes have usually developed a strong commitment to continuing education (Hawes, 1989). In a period of change and development within the NHS, continuing education is perhaps even more important (Collis, 1991). Some authors have stressed the importance of including the technical aspects of care in the continuing education programmes of school nurses. The need to maintain a high level of clinical expertise results from the increased presence of medically complex students in schools (Fegly *et al.*, 1993; Felton and Parsons, 1993). Whatever the level of training or of commitment, it is difficult to see how nurses can adequately meet needs with case loads of the current size.

Expanding aspects of the current job

Some aspects of the current job are visible because they relate to the current concerns of society. They do not have any underlying logic or rationale but demonstrate a widely-held view that certain interventions are needed within schools. The first aspect relates to the recognition of signs and symptoms and covers drugs and alcohol, anorexia and child neglect or abuse. Another expanding area relates to the caring role, and covers the clinical needs of children with chronic illnesses, the immediate needs of those who are injured, including those injured in school games and athletics, and also the care of pregnant teenagers. The role as screener or immuniser has seen several new angles. Another development is that of researcher/epidemiologist.

Recognition of signs

One of the problem areas for schools and for nurses is that of drugs and alcohol. There are problems of recognition of signs and symptoms of substance abuse, and a general lack of knowledge of how to manage overdose situations. One aid may be a nursing assessment tool which has been developed to identify students who may be using drugs or alcohol. It may identify students who need immediate medical care as well as those who are impaired by substance abuse but medically stable (Cromwell and LeMoine, 1992). Following a survey of cases referred to a regional poisons centre from schools, it appears that school nurses are not well prepared to recognise problems and are inadequately trained to deal with them (Perry *et al.*, 1992). Another problem area for early recognition is that of eating disorders. Anorexia nervosa is identified with increasing frequency amongst adolescents. School nurses can play an important role in primary, secondary and tertiary prevention. Connolly and Corbett

(1990) propose a case-management role for school nurses and consider that school nurses are uniquely placed to address these disorders. The school physician and the school nurse have special opportunities to detect situations of distress in children (Mantz, 1990). The importance of recognising neglect and intervening with these children's families is an essential element of the role of the school nurse (Reis, 1993).

The caring role

Given the increasing number of children with chronic diseases who are in mainstream schools, it is inevitable that the school nurse will increasingly be involved in supporting their medical needs (Repetto and Hoeman, 1991; Joachim, 1989). Some of the conditions are common; for example, asthma. In an intervention study, Hill *et al.* (1991) set out to determine whether a programme based on existing school and community resources could reduce school absence and improve participation in games lessons and sport in children with unrecognised asthma. Teachers were given education on asthma by the school nurses. Other conditions are rarely seen. Cooper (1989) gave an account of the key role that a school nurse provided for a child with a tracheostomy. One of the many issues that school nurses have to face is that of school-age pregnancy which may involve providing antenatal support to young women at school (Chen *et al.*, 1991).

Screening/immunisation

The literature on the role of the school nurse in relation to immunisation will have to be rewritten following their involvement in the mass measles/rubella campaign in November 1994. Anecdotal evidence suggests that school nurses were central to the programme's overall success. Their role in Canada's largest mass immunisation programme has been described by Bernatchez *et al.* (1993). In schools in North America, nurses play a pivotal role in the ascertainment of the appropriate immunisation status of school children. One of the long-standing issues has been whether a doctor should or should not be present at the time nurses give immunisations (Saffin, 1992). On the screening side, there have been calls for the application of many different screening programmes, few of which have properly assessed their effectiveness.

One recent proposal suggested the school nurse has a role in the detection of abnormal colour perception and in the education and counselling of the affected student, parents and teachers (Evans, 1992).

Researcher and epidemiologist

Nurses are, in some cases, the developing focus for research into the health status and health problems of children. Several authors now see them as a key part of the research team. If school nurses become involved in systematic measurement, it raises the question of the reliability and validity of such measurements (Kelsall and Watson, 1990; Parker, 1992; Cotterill *et al.*, 1993; Majrowski *et al.*, 1994).

Health promotion opportunities

In this final section, consideration will be given to the current role of school nurses in health promotion, and the constraints and opportunities to enlarging that role. The opportunities are extensive for the introduction of health promotion as part of the curriculum. For school nurses to develop as the key figures in the school health service, they must broaden their role as health educators and health promoters (Johnson, 1991). It has been widely recognised that teachers do not feel adequately prepared for sex-education programmes. This issue was studied by Jackson (1989) in a study of all of the secondary schools and four special schools in Halton. Given teachers' general discomfiture, it is even more important that school nurses should be well trained and comfortable in discussing sex education. An important issue is at what age sex education in schools should begin. The prevailing view is that education about AIDS and HIV should start in primary school if positive attitudes and behaviour are to be effectively encouraged (Mole, 1991).

One aspect of health promotion is the provision of information. This applies both to the children themselves, and also to parents. Patterson (1990) described how a request for health information from mothers of young children led to a regular discussion group and a successful partnership between the school nurse and her health visitor colleagues.

In the current climate of health service market orientation purchasers are being required to separate the specification of health promotion and health education from its actual delivery. The actual organisation of health promotion differs in different districts. In some it is an integral part of the district public health department; in others it is quasi independent; and in yet others it is a part of, or an entirely separate, legal entity. Examples include being part of a Trust or local authority. Health educators have usually worked a combination of direct contact with individuals (children) and indirect contact through other health and educational professionals. In many districts, the absolute size of the health promotion and health education group is so small that it is difficult for them to function successfully even if they only aspire to an indirect role. For this role to be successful, health educators must develop close working relationships with other health professionals. An obvious candidate is the school nurse. They recognise that opportunity alone in schools is not enough but needs to be accompanied by well-developed programmes and policies. In many districts the relationship between health promotion specialist and school nurse is close and contacts are frequent. In some, substantial time has been set aside for the development of the school nurse role.

Health promotion constraints

Constraints remain much as before. They depend to some extent on the imagination of the school nurse to accept the challenges that others are grasping. They depend largely on the climate of health service reforms which have seen a substantial increase in the monitoring of activity and an increase in the political importance of acute hospital activity. The emphasis here is on waiting lists, hospital beds and day-case surgery. Again, the school is relatively invisible and the methods of monitoring community nursing service in general and school nursing activities in particular is poorly developed. When purchasers demand cost improvements in the budgets of community services this may well mean a reduction in the number of school nurses. It requires a strong school nursing service to survive within a Community Trust, and a strong public health department at purchaser level to advocate its survival. In future, when GPs have an increasing say in how the health authority budget is to be spent they are likely to be less sympathetic than those who currently take decisions about financial allocation. Given the preference for 'market testing' of health and social services and for the movement into the independent sector of much of health and educational provision, it is likely that school health services and school nursing services will be casualties in their current form.

If the next decade is to see the survival of the school nursing service, it will be because of the recognition of its value by children and their parents. Although at present their voices have only a minor influence on such policy decisions it is not inconceivable that these voices will become louder. If lessons from the United States teach us anything, it is that the school nursing service will disappear in many places. Recreating it may not be easy. With that in mind, and more in the spirit of conviction politics than rational argument, the challenge for school nurses is to grasp the many opportunities that exist. They must so enthuse the school system, children, parents and governors, that those who take funding decisions will acknowledge the system's high profile and potential worth. The fact that the demonstration of effectiveness may be difficult in the short or medium term should not detract from the fact that there are many opportunities for instant feedback and visible success.

References

Adams, C. (1990). Perceptions of the comprehensive-based school nurse. *Health Visitor*, *63*(3), 90–92.

Adams, C. (1991). An analysis of school nurse leadership styles. *Journal of School Nursing* (April), *7*(2), 22–25.

Adams, C. E. (1992). Identification and recovery of co-dependent school nurses. *Journal of School Nursing* (April), *8*(2), 14–15, 18–19.

Bagnall, P. (1989). School nursing: time to face the future. *Health Visitor* (July), *62*(7), 224.

Bagnall, P. (1991). School nursing comes of age. *Health Visitor*, *64*(5), 146–147.

Bax, M. & Whitmore, K. (1991). Every child should have one. *Health Visitor* (May), *64*(5), 157–159.

Bays, C. T. (1991). The school nurse: enhancing professional recognition. Journal of School Nursing (Oct), *7*(3), 18–20, 22–24.

Bernatchez, M., Grakist, D., Lachance, M., Marks, S., Rodney, J. & Traversy Wong, M. (1993). Operation Meningo: public health nurses' role in Canada's largest mass immunisation program. *Journal of School Health* (Dec), *63*(10), 434–437.

Bolton, P. (1994). School entry screening by the school nurse. *Health Visitor* (April), *67*(4), 135–136.

Chen, S. P., Fitzgerald, M. C., DeStefano, L. M. & Chen, E. H. (1991). *Public Health Nurse* (Dec), *8*(4), 212–218.

Cohen, P. (1994). The role of the school nurse in providing sex education. *Nursing Times* (June 8–14), *90*(23), 36–38.

Collis, J. (1991). Education. What school nurses want. *Health Visitor* (May), *64*(5), 160–161.

Connolly, C. & Corbett, D. P. (1990). Eating disorders: a framework for school nursing initiatives. *Journal of School Health* (October), *60*(8), 401–405.

Cooper, H. (1989). Tracheostomy care in an educational setting. *Health Visitor* (November), *62*, 348–349.

Cotterill, A. M., Majrowski, W. H., Hearn, S. J., Jenkins, S. & Savage, M. O. (1993). Assessment of the reliability of school nurse height measurements in an inner city population. *Child Care Health Development* (May–June), *19*(3), 159–165.

Cromwell, P. & LeMoine, A. (1992). Identifying substance use: an assessment tool for the school nurse. *Journal of School Nursing* (October), *8*(3), 6–10, 12, 14–15.

Cutting, E. & Fahey, W. (1988). What parents expect from primary school health services. *Health at School* (June), *2*(9), 269–270.

Czajka, L. & George, T. B. (1991). School nursing is alive and well in Kalamazoo, thanks to Nazareth College nursing students. *Public Health Nurse*, *8*, 3, 166–169.

Doggett, M. A., Faulkner, A., Farrow, S. & Shelley, A. (1992). School nurses: constraints and opportunities for the future. *Journal of the Royal Society for Health* (April), *112*(2), 84–87.

Dolan, R., Corber, S. & Zacour, R. (1990). A survey of knowledge and attitudes with regard to AIDS among grade 7 and 8 students in Ottawa-Carleton. *Canadian Journal of Public Health* (March–April), *81*(2), 135–138.

Elliott, M., Jones, J. C., Jones, R., Pritchard, V. G. & Robinson, B. E. (1994). An inter-district audit of the school entry medical examination in Cheshire. *Public Health* (May), *108*(3), 203–210.

Evans, A. (1992). Colour vision deficiency – what does it matter? *Journal of School Nursing* (December), *8*(4), 6–10.

Fahey, W. & Cutting, E. (1988). What parents expect from secondary school health services. *Health at School* (June), *3*(9), 272–274.

Fahey, W. & Cutting, E. (1989). What teachers expect from the school health services. *Health at School* (June), *4*(9), 280–282.

Fegly, B. J., Wessel, G. L. & Diehl, B. C. (1993). Clinical continuing education for school nurses. *Journal of School Nursing* (October), *9*(3), 13–14, 16.

Felton, G. M. & Parsons, M. A. (1993). Improving school nursing practice in South Carolina through continuing education. *Journal of School Nursing* (May), *63*(5), 207–209.

Greenhill, E. D. (1979). Perception of the school nurse's role. *Journal of School Health* (September), 368–371.

Hansen, L. (1987). No longer the nit lady. *Nursing Times* (3 June), 30–32.

Harrison, A. & Gretton, J. (1986). School health: the invisible service. In, Health Care UK, an economic, social and policy audit. *Hermitage: Policy Journals*, 25–32.

Hawes, M. (1989). School nursing in Norwich Health Authority. *Health Visitor* (November), *62*(11), 351–352.

Health Visitors Association (1988). *Meeting Schoolchilden's Health Needs*. London: HVA.

Hill, R., Williams, J., Britton, J. & Tattersfield, A. (1991). Can morbidity associated with untreated asthma in primary school children be reduced?: a controlled intervention study. *British Medical Journal*, *303*(6811), 1169–1174.

Houghton, A., Ean, S., Archibal, G., Bradley, O. & Azam, N. (1992). Selective medical examination at school entry: should we do it, and if so how? *Journal of Public Health Medicine* (June), *14*(2), 111–116.

Hunter, A. (1991). A week in the life of Alice Hunter. *Health Visitor* (May), *64*(5), 162–163.

Igoe, J. B. (1994). School nursing. *Nursing Clinics of North America* (September), *29*(3), 443–458.

Jackson, C. (1991). Turning back the clock. *Health Visitor* (May), *64*(5), 148–149.

Jackson, C. (1992). Swings and roundabouts. *Health Visitor* (November), *65*(11), 392–393.

Jackson, D. (1989). Sex education in Halton secondary schools. *Health Visitor* (July), *62*, 219–221.

Joachim, G. (1989). The school nurse as case manager for chronically ill children. Journal of School Health (November), *59*(9), 406–407.

Johnson, J. (1991). Classroom health promotion. *Health Visitor* (May), *64*(5), 152–153.

Jones, M. E. & Clark, D. (1993). What school nurses really do – a study of school nurse utilisation. *Journal of School Nursing* (April), *9*(2), 10–17.

Kelsall, J. E. & Watson, A. R. (1990). Should school nurses measure blood pressure. *Public Health* (May), *104*(3), 191–194.

Kobokovich, L. J. & Bonovich, L. K. (1992). Adolescent pregnancy prevention strategies used by school nurses. *Journal of School Health* (January), *62*(1), 11–14.

Lochhead, E. (1994). Introducing nursery nurses to the school health team. *Health Visitor* (April), *67*(4), 133–134.

Majrowski, W. H., Hearn, S., Rohan, C., Jenkins, S., Cotterill, A. M. & Savage, M. O. (1994). Comparison of school nurse and auxologist height velocity measurements in school children with short stature. *Child Care Health Development* (May–June), *20*(3), 179–183.

Mantz, J. (1990). The school physician and the abused child. *Annals of Pediatrics*, Paris (February), *37*(2), 123–126.

Mattock, C. (1991). Health interviews. Stepping off the medical treadmill. *Health Visitor* (May), *64*(5), 154–156.

Mole, S. (1991). AIDS education in schools. *Health Visitor* (July), *64*(7), 221–222.

National Association of State School Nurse Consultants (1993). A position statement of the National Association of State School Nurse Consultants. Medicaid reimbursement for school nursing services. August 1993. *Journal of School Nursing* (October), *9*(3), 37–39.

Nelson, M. (1989). The changing role of the school nurse within Worcester and District Health Authority. *Health Visitor*, *62*, 349–350.

Orr, J. (1991). Valuing school nurses. *Health Visitor* (May), *64*(5), 147.

Parker, S. H. (1992). The school nurse's role: early detection of growth disorders. *Journal of School Nursing* (October), *8*(3), 30–32, 34, 36–38.

Parsons, M. A. & Felton, G. M. (1992). Role performance and job satisfaction of school nurses. *Western Journal of Nursing Research* (August), *14*(4), 498–511.

Patterson, A. (1990). A school nurse and health visitor working together as health educators. *Health Visitor* (November), *63*(11), 391.

Perry, P. A., Dean, B. S. & Krenzelok, E. P. (1992). A regional poison centre's experience with poisoning exposures occurring in schools. *Veterinary and Human Toxicology* (April), *34*(2), 148–151.

Primary Health Care Group (1988). *Changing School Health Service*. King's Fund Centre for Health Services Development, January 1988. London: King's Fund Centre.

Reis, M. (1993). The neglected pre-school child. *Canadian Nurse* (February), *89*(2), 42–45.

Repetto, M. A., Hoeman, S. P. (1991). A legislative perspective on the school nurse and education for children with disabilities in New Jersey. *Journal of School Nursing* (November), *61*(9), 388–391.

Roberts, P. J. (1993). The school leaver medical: and evaluation. *Public Health* (March), *107*(2), 113–116.

Saffin, K. (1992). School nurses immunising without a doctor present. *Health Visitor* (November), *65*(11), 394–396.

Staunton, P. (1983). Images of the primary school nurse. *Nursing Times* (31 August), 49–52.

Thompson, J. (1989). School health services in the United States: a view from the United Kingdom. *Journal of School Health* (August), *59*(6), 243–245.

Thurber, F., Berry, B. & Cameron, M. E. (1991). The role of school nursing in the United States. *Journal of Pediatric Health Care* (May–June), *5*(3), 135–140.

Turner, T. (1994). A message for Mrs Bottomley. *Health Visitor* (April), *67*(4), 121–122.

Vine, P. (1991). Ninety nine and counting. *Health Visitor* (May), *64*(5), 150–151.

While, A. E. & Barriball, K. L. (1993). School nursing: history, present practice and possibilities reviewed. *Journal of Advanced Nursing* (August), *18*(8), 1202–1211.

Williamson, T. (1992). Health care interviews by school nurses. *Health Visitor* (November), *65*(11), 402–404.

Yates, S. R. (1992). The school nurse's role: early intervention with preschool children. *Journal of School Nursing* (December), *8*(4), 30–36.

14 Health promotion in a youth work setting

Miriam Jackson

With the publication of *The Health of the Nation* (Department of Health, 1992), the Government identified specific health targets for children and young people. These included reductions in cigarette smoking, under-age pregnancy, obesity and suicides among young men. Effective youth service provision already exists in each of these areas and could be enhanced and extended to help meet these targets. Frequently, however, the role and contribution which youth service organisations can make to young peoples health, are overlooked.

Youth work is largely concerned with the informal education of young people, as individuals and as groups, and particularly but not exclusively within the 13-19 age range, a time of critical transition from adolescence to adulthood when they are perhaps more urgently in need of knowledge and information about matters which affect their mental, emotional and physical health. As such, it is a primary location for health education.

Youth work takes place in a variety of settings. These settings include local authority youth clubs and centres, detached work projects, girls groups, sports clubs, youth advice and information centres; also in voluntary organisation groups such as the Scouts, Guides, PHAB clubs (physically handicapped and able-bodied), youth theatres and many other single-focus activity groups. These places are young peoples spaces, their territory where they feel safe and operate on their own terms with adults they know and trust. Additionally, and of enormous significance, is the fact that young people participate in these activities voluntarily, choosing to attend rather than being compelled to do so, as with school and formal education settings.

This combination of factors makes youth work perhaps unique in educational terms. Young people are centre stage, and feel safe with their peers and with trusted adults, in their own free time, without external pressures. Such a ready established setting offers tremendous potential for health promotion. Used well and sensitively, youth work presents opportunities for educational work with young people often impossible to recreate elsewhere.

Some regional and district health authorities have recognised the

157

potential impact that progressive and innovative youth projects can make, and have provided funding. The Health Line project, for example, in Liverpool, aims to raise young peoples awareness of health issues, provides advice, helps people to access local health services, supports peer education programmes and provides training for workers (Merseyside Youth Association, 88 Shiel Road, Liverpool). Similarly, 'Court in the Act', a drink-driving awareness-raising programme involves the local police in North Yorkshire (North Yorkshire Community Education Service, County Hall, Northallerton); and a peer health project in Portslade led to a GP practice nurse being integrated into youth club sessions to offer a friendly face, health advice and a gateway to local GPs (Portslade Village Centre, Portslade, East Sussex). These projects offer practical examples of provision which works, and of dynamic partnerships between health professionals and the youth service.

Accessing young people

Generally, there is ignorance among health authorities about the existence of the youth service and its potential in promoting healthy young people. As a result, much health focused youth work continues unaided and unrecognised. *The Health of the Nation* is now shaping thinking, and strategies for health and partnerships and healthy alliances are being promoted. Not only can the youth service make a very real contribution in delivery terms, it is also capable of providing expert advice and guidance at the planning and policy level.

A recent Government survey by the Office of Population Censuses and Surveys (OPCS) included questions on young peoples involvement with the youth service. Out of a total of 3700 young people contacted in late 1993 and early 1994, this survey showed that 20 per cent of young people aged between 13 and 19 currently participate in youth service activities (Department for Education, 1995). Translated to a national scale, that is something in the order of 840 000 young people and does not include the millions of under elevens involved in the junior wings of uniformed organisations or junior youth clubs.

The researchers say the figures suggest that the youth service reaches 63 per cent of young people at some time during their teenage years. A conservative estimate would be some 2.7 million. While cynics might think the OPCS used a very loose definition of youth service participation, the researchers say that their sample was broadly constructed to include those using the service randomly or intensively. Of those aged between 11 and 25 who use the service, the majority seems to use it a lot, some 1.13 million at least once each week.

Surely a service that can demonstrate the voluntary engagement of such numbers of young people at times generally regarded in health terms as important, and when lifestyle habits and behaviour are being established, should not be overlooked when health promotion initiatives are being formulated and healthy alliances promoted. The youth service, voluntary and statutory, is making a real contribution to the lives of a lot of young people, and policymakers would be advised to take note if they are genuinely committed to improving services for young people and meeting Government targets.

The Health of the Nation targets for young people

Youth service provision can clearly demonstrate work specific to the Governments identified health targets for young people. For example, 42nd Street, a project in Manchester, works specifically on issues of mental health, stress, break down and suicide in young people particularly from ethnic minority backgrounds (for further details contact 42nd Street, Ground Floor, Lloyds House, 22 Lloyd Street, Manchester and see the 42nd Street Annual Report, 1994). To date, the project has promoted a greater understanding and awareness of mental health issues, helped young people to develop coping mechanisms and created links with specialist mental health provision. Additionally, it has worked with other agencies and developed materials and helped train others. Youth services in Hereford and Worcester and in Rochdale are seeking advice from 42nd Street while attempting to set up similar projects to meet identified needs for which no other services are available locally. Funded for three years from a youthwork development grant supportive of innovative and responsive youth work, it will be interesting to see what funding 42nd Street secures beyond this point. The Governments target for reducing cigarette smoking among the under-16s, is a cut in the present figures by 50 per cent. So far, Government initiatives and advertising campaigns would seem to have had little influence on young peoples smoking patterns which 1992 figures show remain virtually unchanged since 1986, at 10 per cent (Royal College of Physicians, 1992). Clearly, more sophisticated methods of influencing teenagers and young people need to be found to tackle the sense of rebellion, maturity and sophistication felt by young smokers.

Youth service approaches include work around self-image and peer group pressure and conformity, as well as specific information on the effects of smoking on health and fitness rather than anti-smoking rhetoric. In Rotherham, the High Energy Health initiative views smoking through a more general approach to fitness and well-being using smoke analysers, dance and exercise, as well as discussion to explore issues around smoking and health and fitness, particularly with young women (for further details contact Rotherham Health Promotion, 1/2 Chatham Villas, Chatham Street, Rotherham). The project, which is funded by health promotion and tours local youth clubs, has attracted a high involvement from young women.

Youth provision until recently usually tolerated smoking for fear of discouraging young peoples participation. Now the picture is very different, with many youth projects designated as smoke free by· young people themselves. Youth workers have provided information, encouraged discussions and facilitated young peoples consideration of the issues themselves. Very often under these circumstances smoking has been limited or banned altogether, perhaps indicating that when given responsibility and autonomy many young people will act with maturity.

Peer education initiatives

Peer education is recognised as an important strategy in working with young people. We all share information with and gain experience from peers, and young people are no exception. Indeed, as their dress codes demonstrate, peer influence is extremely high. The youth service has long recognised and exploited this informal method of education either in group settings, in young leader and helper schemes, and in more formalised situations where young people receive specific training and support and then share their knowledge with other young people.

Many youth service projects exist where groups of young people are working with their peers on health-related issues. In Norfolk, for example, a young mums group leads sessions in local schools on the realities of teenage pregnancy, another Government target. (Further details can be obtained from the Young Mums Education Project, The Risebrow Centre, Chantry Road, Norwich). The Health Education Authority (HEA) is funding a Health in Clubs project based at ten clubs throughout the country and managed by Youth Clubs UK, a national voluntary youth organisation. Young people are recruited and trained using a specially developed peer education framework after which they are encouraged and supported to establish various local peer learning groups facilitated by themselves. Most, though not all, are focused on sexual health issues, with one group concentrating on the sexual health needs of gay young men while another looks at the needs of young women.

This is the only national initiative specifically focused on health education through youth work. No funding has been made available to explore the implications of *The Health of the Nation* or its targets for the youth service, or to help the youth service further develop its health education role. Naturally, much is being done locally, but with encouragement, coordination and dissemination from the centre much more could be done to enhance the contribution of youth work to health education.

A healthy schools initiative has been developed by the HEA, but there is no similar healthy youth club initiative (NHS Executive, 1993). Nonetheless, some youth work projects have seized upon the idea as one which can stimulate effective work with members, but without support, funding or recognition of the work that already goes on. This is not a productive way of securing the best contribution to young peoples health education from a service already well placed to help. And with the imminent funding cuts to the HEA, its potential to pioneer and promote innovative health education initiatives of any kind will almost certainly be abandoned.

The youth work contribution

The growth and development of health promotion as a distinct profession has in some instances reduced youth workers inclusion of health education in the curriculum. The presence of the health education specialists has often meant youth workers deferring to these professionals and feeling de-skilled and demotivated alongside them. Health education and health promotion specialists, however, recognise the distinct advantages youth workers have when it comes to educative work with young people. Youth workers already have relationships with young people, meeting with them on their territory and in situations which are relaxed and informal and of the young peoples choosing. This special relationship, coupled with their interpersonal skills, means youth workers are singularly well placed to facilitate effective health education work. While youth workers may not have the specialist health education knowledge base, this can be found or provided at relatively short notice. Establishing relationships of trust and confidence on the other hand is a much lengthier process. Many are now recognising the unique position youth workers occupy and how through working together with health education professionals they can make an impact.

The healthy alliances promoted by *The Health of the Nation* exemplified in youth service and specialist health promotion working together can be seen to achieve more than either could do alone. However, while there is much evidence to support this, there are probably yet more examples of the services working in isolation with little knowledge of and cooperation with one another, or of each striving to produce results which could be gained so much more easily if working together.

In Great Yarmouth and Waveney District Health Authority, for example, an outreach project was established in youth clubs in recognition of the fact that the health authority was not reaching high numbers of young people (Robinson, 1994). Ten sites were selected and health advisers were appointed to each. The advisers, all with a specialist background, facilitated a considerable amount of health promotion work which it is very unlikely would have been addressed in typical youth club situations, or in the traditional sites in which health education officers work.

Some advisers, it has to be admitted, found their working conditions too noisy and smoky, but even such adverse factors were used to advantage. Smoke analysers were taken into clubs to show the affects of smoking, and young people aware generally of smoking being unhealthy were shocked by more specific information on its affects. Other work included health education games and quizzes, group and one-to-one discussions on topics as diverse as skin care, toxic shock syndrome, diet, death and bereavement, homophobia, alcohol, and relationships and sex. Health noticeboards were also set up, and demonstrations carried out on the use of contraceptives, and how to perform breast and testicular self-examinations.

Evaluation of the project, after one year, found that not only had awareness of a wide range of issues been raised, but that young peoples confidence in the health service and knowledge about what it offered had radically increased. Additionally, a small number of specific health problems had been uncovered and referred, and access had been gained to young people who demonstrated behaviour relevant to targets set by *The Health of the Nation* and the health authority. If health authorities are looking to purchase primary preventive health care for young people, such projects would seem to be a good investment.

Most health services for young people are provided alongside those for either adults or children, neither of whose needs young people share. The 1989 Children Act (Department of Health, 1989) emphasises the fact that children and young people have the right to information, consultation and services. This, coupled with *The Health of the Nation* report specifying for the first time targets for healthy young people, should have led to improvements in young peoples health services. The current Government has, however, failed to provide commensurate funding to enable such improvements to be made, and has created a climate in which meeting some of these targets is more difficult. Its refusal, for example, to allow the publication of the HEAs sex-education book recently, and new legislation, has restricted the ability of professionals to provide effective sexual-health education. Statistics from the Netherlands show that the commonly held fear that increased sex education will lead to more teenage pregnancy is unfounded. The Dutch have experienced a decline in teenage pregnancy to 10 per 1000 girls aged 15 to 20 years (Nyman, 1993). The UK, however, has witnessed a rise to 69 per 1000 girls aged 15 to 20 years.

Young people in various surveys have shown that they want access to good information, to counsellors and specialist teachers, as well as settings in which they can discuss sexual matters openly and without fear of judgment. Staff working with young people are convinced of the need for more and better sex education and increased dialogue about feelings, relationships and the affects on the lives of young people if they are to deal with difficult and complicated information and make informed choices and potentially life-changing decisions. The Government has, if anything, facilitated a decrease in both quality and quantity through its legislation and lack of funding.

When asked, young people request services and facilities similar to those provided in most youth clubs and projects - relaxed surroundings, warmth, music and sympathetic listening adults (Wallace, undated). With limited resources, much could be done to meet young peoples needs by merely fully utilising the settings already available and resourcing them to more fully meet the needs young people have identified. If something exists, surely it is more efficient and effective to use that well than establish another provision of broadly similar lines.

Other surveys show that many young people are still not practising safer sex, perhaps because of youthful optimism and resilience, or a blind hope that it will not happen to them (Hurrelmann and Losel, 1990). Much remains to be done here, and attempting to provide what young people themselves are identifying would seem a useful starting point.

Effective youth work practice can also be demonstrated in health related areas outside those set out in *The Health of the Nation*. Low levels of sport and physical activity by young people have also recently become a concern. Team games are to become compulsory within the school curriculum to the great dismay of many young people and their teachers. Many young people freely spend much of their time within their youth projects undertaking some form of physical or sporting activity. Young women who huddle by the side of a hockey or netball pitch will happily dance all night at their youth club. Many turned off by competitive team games will often participate in canoeing or climbing. So much more could be done, however, with increased awareness from workers and recognition from others of the contribution the youth service could make in this respect.

Increasingly, too, these activities are seen not only for their inherent challenges, but also as a way of contributing to a healthy lifestyle and general well-being. Many projects now specifically explore the relationship of sport to fitness and perhaps to body shape and weight. Additionally, clubs offer a variety of sports which are non-competitive yet strenuous and challenging.

Sport in the youth work context once again benefits from participants having free choice regarding participation, and with that comes the challenge for youth workers to ensure a range of physical activities which can be enjoyed by many different individuals. Recently, the measure of 30 minutes of exercise a day was publicised as a health benchmark. Many youth workers may well already provide for this or certainly could do so in the future with little extra effort, being able easily to accommodate anything from roller skating to mountain biking, or dancing to canoeing.

Healthy alliances

In a recent Government Green Paper, *Tackling Drugs Together*, four government departments outlined their joint strategy against drug misuse, drawing attention immediately to their very different starting point from that of the majority of young people (Department for Education, 1994). New money is being found to train teachers to deliver drugs education in schools and to fund ten innovative drug projects. Additionally, the Department for Education is to publish advice on how to teach about drugs, develop drug prevention policies and how to deal with drug-related incidents. Home Office monies will establish 11 local drug action teams and a drugs helpline.

Once again, the youth service contribution is unrecognised, but hopefully the spirit of joint work will be followed through locally and the youth service may be involved in school drug education and in the local action teams. Many specialised projects such as Streetwise in Newcastle, a drop-in advice and guidance service for young people on drug and alcohol-related issues, have a history of making an impact with young people and could be further developed and pursued elsewhere (for further details contact Streetwise, 35–37 The Groat Market, Newcastle upon Tyne, and see their Annual Report 1992/93).

Questions must be asked as to why young people find the proposition of taking drugs to be an exciting one. Youth workers recognise that this is because many young people are bored, lack access to leisure facilities and the money to do what they wish. This is coupled with their enthusiasm and energy for something dangerous and stimulating. Here, good youth provision could play a part, and, with extra resources targeted not at the prevention of drug misuse but more positively at providing opportunities for sophisticated, accessible, challenging and enjoyable activities which simultaneously address the need of young people for self-confidence and recognition, many would find drugs a less powerful attraction than at present.

Rave culture has become synonymous with drug taking which has in turn led to the condemnation of raves. In Hartlepool and at a Hinckley leisure centre youth club in Leicestershire, however, drug-free raves have been staged with remarkable success. Many youngsters were pleased that they could attend such an event and stay out overnight dancing with their parents blessing (for further details contact Hartlepool drug and alcohol service, 10 Grange Road, Hartlepool; Health education in youth work, Leicester Community Education Service, County Hall, Glenfield, Leicester). Information about drugs was given out and workers were available to discuss drugs and other issues. For many, it was clear that the highs associated with raves are not about taking drugs, but about fun, friendship, dancing, and being treated like adults. Of course such provision needs to be staffed and paid for, and here once again the potential contribution that youth provision can make needs to be recognised if it is to be funded, and so enabled to make a contribution.

If governments, health authorities and health Trusts are genuinely committed to seeing improvements in primary health care for young people, there is much to be done. Often, identifying action is very difficult but in this case some answers are clear, what is missing is the real commitment to take the question seriously enough. This is not to suggest that the youth service can or indeed should become fundamentally a health education service. However, its contribution to the health education of young people should be recognised by managers and workers within the service, and by funders and others outside the service. Until such recognition is given, good work will continue to be done on an *ad hoc* and individual basis, when so much more is possible.

References

Department for Education (1994). *Tackling Drugs Together: A Consultation Document on a Strategy for England 1995–1998*. London: HMSO.

Department for Education (1995). *Statistical Bulletin 1/95*. London: HMSO.

Department of Health (1992). *The Health of the Nation*. London: HMSO.

Department of Health (1989). *Childrens Act*. London: HMSO.

Hurrelman and Losel (eds) (1990). *Health Hazards in Adolescence*. Berlin: Walter de Gruyter.

NHS Executive (1993). *Priorities and Planning Guidance for the NHS in 1994/95*. London: HMSO.

Nyman, B R. (1993). Going Dutch - a pipe dream. *Family Planning*, 19, 200–203.

Robinson, K. (1994). *Report on Outreach Work Undertaken in Youth Clubs by a Team of Health Advisers*. Great Yarmouth and Waveney District Health Authority: Department of Public Health Medicine.

Royal College of Physicians (1992). *Smoking and the Young*. London: Royal College of Physicians.

Wallace, B. (ed) (undated). *Young People Speak Out About Sex*. Newcastle Health Authority/Newcastle Education Service.

15 *Health promotion in further education*

Ann Payne

Since 1989, the Health Education Authority (HEA), in accordance with the World Health Organisation's 'settings' approach, has sponsored three major projects within the further education (FE) sector. Two of these were national projects which supported a number of colleges in the development of health-related initiatives. The third project was predominantly based in one college, Bournville College of Further Education, and explored a whole college approach to health promotion.

This chapter is based on experience gained from working with colleges in the national projects, that is the *Health in Further Education Project* (1989–1993), and more recently the *Health Promoting College Project* (April 1993–March 1995). The focus of the *Health in Further Education* project was primarily the curriculum and methods of delivery. Colleges were supported in developing initiatives to offer health education to a wider range of students than had traditionally been considered. The emphasis was particularly on the 16–19 age group. However, the success or failure of this approach was found to depend crucially on the quality of management support. The later project, the Health Promoting College project, therefore, had a special emphasis on the involvement of senior management and sought to promote a whole college approach.

Characteristics of further education

The FE sector in England comprises 452 colleges serving a population of almost two million students (1992 figures), representing age groups ranging from 16-year-old school leavers to mature students of 70+ years. From the age of 14, during term time, school students can also attend 'Link' courses at college in preparation for post-statutory education. No other educational institution caters for such a diverse population.

During the decade from 1982 to 1992, the number of 16 year olds participating full-time in further education increased steadily (12 per cent), whilst the number of 18 to 20 year olds rose more steeply (71

167

per cent) and the number of mature students, defined by the Department of Further Education Statistics Bulletin as post-21 year olds, increased quite dramatically (165 per cent). This has inevitably put pressure on college facilities and created accommodation needs.

Although in many other respects similar to schools, FE colleges tend on the whole to be larger institutions, often spread across a number of sites. They not only cater for their local community, but also for students from all parts of the country and from abroad, attracting both young people and experienced adults to specialist courses such as those in maritime navigation, catering and hotel management, the oil industry and so forth.

Prospective FE students may have to compete with many other candidates for a place on courses which are over-subscribed, and they undergo a rigorous written and oral selection process before being accepted. Once enrolled, they can be advised to leave the course or to transfer to a different level, if their attendance and performance fall below the standard required by the certificating body. With retention and completion rates now linked closely to funding, there is increased pressure on the selection process. Ryder and Campbell (1988) stress the need for flexibility, pointing out the difference in previous educational experiences that students will have had, how this affects their learning needs, and the dilemma this may pose for FE colleges which offer narrow schemes of training.

Students may attend an FE college full-time (every day), part-time (a set number of hours each week), on day release (usually one day per week), or for one or two evening classes. So, students are usually in a position to choose whether or not to attend, which course of study to follow, and also whether to remain on that course or leave, if they feel it is not satisfying their needs. College classes, although varying in size according to subject and department, are often larger than those commonly found in extended sixth forms.

Lecturing staff in FE may be employed on full-time permanent contracts, or on part-time, fixed-term contracts, some for as little as two or three hours per week. Most colleges also have a mixture of staff, with subject specialists, recruited from industry and who have not undertaken the Certificate in Education, working alongside qualified and experienced teachers. This tendency to subject specialism may have contributed in the past to a certain insularity in some faculty divisions.

Organisational factors affecting FE

In 1993, FE colleges underwent a major change of status. They became independent, incorporated businesses, funded centrally by the newly established Further Education Funding Council (FEFC). This body both funds the colleges and sets them their broad financial targets. Since 1993, therefore, FE has undergone a period of rapid and sustained change. Many colleges have reorganised, often opting for a flatter management structure, similar to models proposed by Peters (1989). These changes have moved many individuals out of the traditional departmental structure, which although insular created security, into newly-created cross-college roles, such as Quality Manager, or Professional Development Officer. At the same time, new accreditation bodies have introduced substantial curriculum change, and an emphasis on processes such as the accreditation of prior learning has created intense demands, alongside continuing problems with securing progression for students into higher education.

The number of teaching hours for courses has been reduced by up to 38 per cent in some cases, resulting in lecturers acquiring responsibility for additional classes, with the resultant increased workload, marking and student support. At the same time, students have been given greater responsibility for their own learning, with increased private study time. Class sizes have been increasing, and with an expansion target recently introduced by the Further Education Funding Council of 25 per cent over three years, this trend will continue. This is despite the fact that many classrooms are small and already overcrowded, with inadequate seating and insufficient resources. Staff feel that, even though they are dealing with steadily increasing student numbers, with less time and fewer resources, they are still expected to improve examination results and pass rates.

Such rapid and extensive innovation appears sometimes to have reached the point where change results in immobilisation, and a feeling among staff that there is no way they can take on anything additional. There is no time to reflect on the potential benefits of a new initiative, or how it might contribute to what they are already attempting to achieve. Managers in FE find themselves having to make decisions and implement strategies which are externally imposed by the FEFC, ones which they perhaps do not fully support themselves. Staff allocate them with the blame for unpopular policies, without realising the dilemmas which managers face. One of the issues causing great difficulty in some colleges is the requirement for staff to sign new contracts of employment. This is a divisive issue, and some staff have signed and others have not; there may be calls for industrial action. To survive and flourish in this confusing climate, colleges need to match the efficiency of their private sector competitors in the provision of training and development, while at the same time maximising their effectiveness as centres of learning for both young people and adults.

The health promoting college project

The introduction of the two-year, national Health Promoting College Project in April 1993 coincided with the move to incorporation, and therefore in theory appeared timely. This project was designed to encourage interested colleges to embrace the concept of becoming health promoting institutions, so as to meet the needs of their college community. The project was underpinned by the practical experience of the two earlier projects, and supported by a helpful, associated publication from the HEA, *The Health Promoting College* (O'Donnell and Gray, 1993). If successfully adopted, it was envisaged that the project approach to health promotion might well help attract and retain students, contribute to the college's independent image, and provide the college with a clear message for its potential market.

As mentioned earlier in the chapter, past experience with the two previous FE projects had clearly indicated the importance of active support from senior management, if the initiative was to survive beyond the timescale of the project and become fully embedded in the institution. For this reason, the project targeted senior managers, and started by consulting with a group of invited Principals, in order to seek advice on strategy and approach. Based on this meeting, the following strategy was affected during year one, April 1993 to March 1994.

Initially, the project sought to reach the network of college managers through channels established by the FEFC. This, however, proved to be a slow and much more complicated process than was first thought. Publicity was therefore circulated direct to all 452 colleges in England, informing them of the HEA's imminent publication of *The Health Promoting College*, and inviting senior managers to one of four regional one-day launches.

Contact was established with the General Secretary of the Association of Principals of Colleges (APC), and through him with the chairperson of the six English branches of the association. Publicity material was distributed to all members of the organisation and short presentations were made at three branch meetings. One problem here was the over-full agenda of each branch, which made it difficult to allocate time to the project even when there was an interest.

A series of three regional one-day launches was held in Spring 1994, at which college decision makers had the opportunity to review the publication, to meet practitioners who had put health promotion strategies into effect, and to develop an action plan. One thing which interested the managers who attended, was the model adapted from O'Donnell and Gray (1993) which provides a framework for development with four key institutional determinants, the institution, the environment, the curriculum and relationships (see *Figure 15.1*).

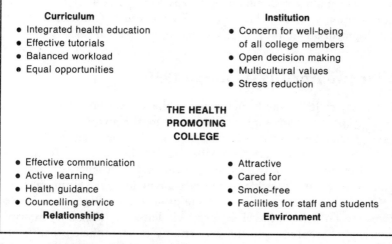

Curriculum
- Integrated health education
- Effective tutorials
- Balanced workload
- Equal opportunities

Institution
- Concern for well-being of all college members
- Open decision making
- Multicultural values
- Stress reduction

THE HEALTH PROMOTING COLLEGE

- Effective communication
- Active learning
- Health guidance
- Councelling service

Relationships

- Attractive
- Cared for
- Smoke-free
- Facilities for staff and students

Environment

Source: adapted from O'Donnell and Gray (1993)

Figure 15.1 *The health promoting college – framework for development*

This model not only offers colleges a framework within which to identify examples of their current good practice, but also provides a structure for illuminating those areas which may need further consideration if adopting a whole-college approach. For example, the health promoting college is one that plans its activities so as to minimise stress and provide support for people. If stress is thought to be a specific health issue within the college community this may be addressed under one or more of the four key determinants.

The initiative may focus on *the institution,* by helping managers to clarify their beliefs and values, consider the impact of different styles of management and promote a clear process of meaningful consultation in the development and implementation of policy. Or it may be that environmental factors are considered the most obvious starting point. A college may wish to make *the environment* more client-friendly and welcoming, perhaps by making greater use of colour, plants, notice boards and displays of student work; or maybe by ensuring there are clear direction signs, or trying to create more quiet space for individual study. Alternatively, health promoting *relationships* may be encouraged by an initiative that considers the need for adequate levels of staffing and resources, the fair distribution of routine and innovative tasks, and the provision of support networks, including counselling services, for staff and students. The most obvious starting point for some colleges will be *the curriculum,* where there may be much good practice already in evidence. This might include extending and enhancing the personal tutorial system to make health promotion available to all students, and the provision of staff development and appropriate resources in support of this.

Year two April 1994–March 1995

For many colleges, the launch acted as the springboard they had been looking for, and with support from their local network they elected to develop and implement their action plan with only minimal contact from the project. Others found that due to the effects of reorganisation, lack of support from management and colleagues, or low staff morale, it was not possible to embrace a new initiative at the time.

Given the limited resources of the project, all colleges were offered access to on-going general support, via letter or telephone; information about resources; and the opportunity to share their progress at a regional network meeting towards the end of the spring term, 1995. Eighteen colleges were also offered supplementary support, consisting of several days of project team time which could be used as the college deemed appropriate, to aid achievement of their action plan.

Support requested by colleges

During the period of sustained consultancy and support, colleges called on the project to provide the following: presentations to senior management groups, and/or multi-disciplinary groups to help establish a shared vision of a health promoting college; work with managers and key staff towards the development of a health promotion policy or statement; consultation with working parties to develop an action plan and explore the best ways of implementing it; and delivery of staff development workshops for multi-disciplinary groups, to address specific health issues within the college community, for example, stress management and coping with change.

Attention was given to evaluating the project throughout by use of questionnaires and selective interviews. The results of these evaluations suggest a number of interesting points. For example, colleges appear to be interpreting the recent 'settings' approach to health promotion in two different ways:

1. The college as a setting which offers health promoting activities – where there is a concentration on curriculum initiatives; the provision of updated health issues information via Student Services; support given to national health promotion days, for example World AIDS Day; and promotion of health through various awareness-raising 'Fairs'.

2. The college as a health promoting setting, where everything about the setting is explored to try to develop a health promoting focus – the whole ethos; the democratic process; management style and values. This approach has to be management led as stated by Baric (1994, p. 200).

> The switch from problems to setting has produced a new set of partners for people engaged in health promotion and health education. These new partners are the members of the management team in the 'setting'. They are the main decision makers, in a position to declare their setting as a health promoting setting.

However, this appears to be a much more nebulous concept, and it is not easy for managers to get a clear vision of what is entailed. They are unsure of how exactly to put a whole college approach into effect. Theoretically, the words sound convincing, but to achieve practical action they need to be translated into clear, concise guidelines.

Similarly, the holistic approach to health and well-being presented some difficulties when compared with the sharper focus of the medical model. Ensuring that opportunities were available to all students to tackle issues such as problem-solving, assertiveness, stress management, dealing with conflict, and negotiating successfully, at a time when course hours were being reduced, could present practical problems. These issues were overcome in some colleges by involving committed staff in piloting the promotion of positive health through the college-wide tutorial system.

Colleges need and appreciate personal support to help them determine an initiative which is appropriate to their college, and to spread the news of good practice from other institutions. Rather than a document or a directive, what they chiefly need is face-to-face assistance.

Another issue concerns how to recognise achievement in promoting health. Some colleges are seeking an award system, like for example the *Investor in People* award, which can act as an incentive to their efforts. Other colleges see this as anathema. The award contradicts all that they are trying to achieve in health promotion, since they believe that it is the process and quality of experience which is important, and not the award at the end.

Those colleges who have been most successful in pursuing a whole college approach are institutions which have managed to link the project with existing, stated priorities for management, such as an *Investors in People* commitment. Promotion of one issue by linking it with another has been the subject of attention in the field of social policy-making elsewhere, for example in Hall *et al.* (1978).

Finally, wherever colleges are starting from in their move towards becoming more health promoting, whether it is with a single curriculum issue or with a wider college approach, a high proportion of them are identifying stress as a major factor needing to be addressed.

Who should be involved?

Undoubtedly, as with any new initiative, it is important to involve people who have a high degree of knowledge and understanding of the innovation, and who are actively motivated to support it. It is also crucial to involve those who have the power both to make and implement decisions, and to allocate funding and resources, as advocated by Elliott-Kemp (1982).

Who should be involved will depend on the 'settings' approach chosen by an institution. A college taking the narrower approach will tend to allocate responsibility for the health promotion initiative to a single individual, and other individuals in the college will tend to disregard the initiative. On the other hand, for the institution choosing the broad approach under the leadership of the management, literally everyone in the college must be involved.

Benefits identified by the colleges

Colleges reported that they found the project useful as a catalyst to their own ideas and plans. It provided them with a focus and a framework within which to act. In addition, the opportunity to meet and share ideas with colleagues from other colleges was valued. It was helpful, too, to learn what was happening elsewhere, and to participate in the spread of good practice. In many colleges, health promotion has declined as a priority, and has ceased to be in the forefront of people's minds. The visits of an external consultant helped bring health back to the top of college agendas. Finally college staff appreciated the effectiveness of the project in spreading the word about health promotion to their management teams.

Future support

In considering the future for health promotion in FE, it is important to recognise the difficulties which colleges have been facing since 1993, and to understand the concerns and priorities discussed earlier. Undoubtedly, some colleges have successfully emerged from the period of expansion and rapid change which followed incorporation and may now be in a position to implement health promotion. Managers and staff welcome the support given by external health professionals and are keen to identify how a whole college approach can be promoted. They may need help to determine how becoming a health promoting institution can underpin the developments which are already proceding within the college, and how health promoting systems and practices can bring benefits for students and staff.

References

Baric, L. (1994) *Health promotion and health education. Module 2: The organisational model.* Cheshire: Barns.

Elliott-Kemp, J. (1982). *Managing Organisational Change.* Sheffield: Pavic Publications.

Hall, P., Land, H., Parker, R. & Webb, A. (1978). *Change, Choice and Conflict in Social Policy.* London: Heinemann.

O'Donnell, T. & Gray, G. (1993). *The Health Promoting College.* London: Health Education Authority.

Peters, T. (1989). *Thriving on Chaos.* London: Pan Books.

Ryder, J. & Campbell, L. (1988). *Balancing Acts.* London: Routledge.

Voluntary

16 *The voluntary setting and its contribution to health promotion*

Yvonne Anderson and Zoë Heritage

This chapter will focus on the main functions of voluntary agencies working in the health promotion field. The classification used describes pressure groups, service providers, information services, community and self-help groups. Most voluntary organisations, however, undertake a number of functions; for example, the National Childbirth Trust works with the Department of Health, organises a self-help network and is active in educating the public. A case study of Victim Support will be described to illustrate some of the ways in which a particular voluntary organisation can contribute to health promotion.

What is the nature of the voluntary setting?

Perhaps the most striking feature of the voluntary setting is its great diversity. It ranges from one unpaid person working from a living room to multi-million pound organisations using highly professional, paid staff. There is no universal definition of a voluntary organisation, but a working definition might include the following characteristics:

- Independent beginnings;
- Self-governing structures;
- Independence from other bodies;
- Surpluses not distributed for profit;
- Worthwhile purposes, increased morality.

These characteristics have been summed up by Knight (1993) as a form of energy stemming from free will, having moral purpose and undertaken in a spirit of independence.

Perri 6 (1991) offers a definition framework in which the narrow voluntary sector includes voluntary organisations and charities, but not the non-profit making organisations such as trade unions, political parties, sports clubs and trade associations. For the purposes of this

179

chapter, the voluntary sector will be taken as the narrow voluntary sector.

In terms of sheer numbers the voluntary sector makes a substantial contribution to the field of health and social welfare. Estimates vary as to the size of the voluntary sector in the UK, as there are difficulties in obtaining statistics on very small local groups and on groups which are not registered as charities. Perri 6 and Fieldgrass (1992) state that the voluntary sector houses around 2 million people and gives formal advice to about 350 000 people every day.

Meeting health needs

The role of the voluntary setting in health promotion cannot be discussed without some appraisal of the statutory agencies. Clearly, if health is understood as something more than just the absence of disease, then many statutory agencies can be seen to play a role in health promotion, whether they provide housing, amenities, residential care or a variety of other services. However, the key player in the field is the National Health Service. In the final analysis, voluntary organisations come about initially in response to a need. Given the proliferation of voluntary organisations in the 1980s, it would appear in line with popular belief that the NHS is not meeting all health needs. Seedhouse (1994, p. 31) suggests that within the NHS there are three main, complementary definitions of health need; which are, the supply or benefit definition, the ill-health definition and the normative definition. All three, he asserts, offer support to the others, so that they are inseparable and '...each is deeply orthodox, protecting and preserving the current state of the NHS, whatever it is at a particular time'.

In other words, the NHS has a self-serving mechanism for the assessment and meeting of health needs. A more simple analysis would stress that there are finite resources with which to run the NHS and that these, set against ever increasing expectations and longer life expectancy, lead to greater health needs which cannot realistically be met.

The NHS may fail to meet health needs in other ways. Seedhouse (*ibid*, p. 9) describes how '...nurses seek to advocate on behalf of the patients but are often prevented from doing so by tight staffing levels and – not uncommonly – by resistance from others with different priorities'. Patients (or clients) of the NHS may also need a more holistic service than that which is currently offered within the confines of a large state bureaucracy.

A recent collaborative venture between statutory and voluntary organisations in Thamesdown identified the health needs of a large group of residents of local neighbourhoods. The residents themselves prioritised needs connected with better safety and security, cleaner streets and decent housing. Whilst many of the identified needs could be partly met by the statutory sector, it is likely that voluntary organisations will play a key role, and the residents themselves gave priority to the need for more self-help and volunteers in the community (Priority Focus 1994).

Diversity in the voluntary sector: the example of victim support

Given the diversity of human needs, it follows that the voluntary sector will be wide ranging. In the top ten charities, ranked by income, Barnardo's spent £52 million on child care in 1991, having a special interest in children and their families affected by HIV and AIDS, homelessness, child abuse and in community support for children. In contrast, the residents associations which characterise many of our larger towns have very limited funding, often from the local council, and may be run from someone's house, relying entirely on volunteers and with no paid staff. The first example of Barnardo's is perhaps quite straightforwardly related to health and welfare. However, if a holistic concept of health is adopted, then, at the other end of the spectrum, even residents associations may be making a positive contribution to health promotion, in influencing safety and cleanliness of the immediate environment and in contributing to people's sense of community.

Similarly, Victim Support is an organisation not overtly concerned with health, but it plays an important, if subtle health promotion role, both for clients and for volunteers. Victim Support began in Bristol in 1974, as a 6-month needs-assessment project. To date, there are about 370 schemes in England and Wales alone and many others in Scotland, Ireland, other European countries, the USA and Australia. The National Association of Victim Support is based in London and from here the guidelines, policy and codes of practice relating to the running of local schemes are issued.

Local schemes may cover an entire county or, more usually, a town or district within a county, for example, Greater Manchester has 13 separate schemes, whilst Hampshire has ten and Wiltshire just one, covering the whole county from a central base. Funding for schemes comes mainly from the national office, which secures its finances from the Home Office and often from local authorities. However, like all voluntary organisations in today's climate, schemes have to conduct their own fund-raising activities, in order to continue to provide their services and to develop beyond minimum requirements.

The scope for health promotion

Voluntary organisations have a variety of functions, some having a single function, but others, more usually, having two or more functions. The majority of voluntary organisations act as *service providers*. Many voluntary organisations provide practical services which can range from delivering a meal, listening to someone's distressed telephone call, to giving full-time residential care to a terminally-ill person. These services are needed because the statutory authorities cannot, for a variety of reasons provide the service themselves. In some instances, voluntary organisations have become the recognised experts in a particular field; for example, St John's Ambulance, or the hospice movement. The service offered by Victim Support is quite specialised and has an important, if indirect, effect on the health of clients. Any victim of crime experiences loss and change, from the seemingly trivial loss of a few garden tools in a garden shed theft, through to the most profound sense of personal loss associated with serious crime, such as rape or murder. Murray-Parkes (1993) has proposed three factors related to life change, which commonly precede mental illness. He claims that the most dangerous life-change events are those that, firstly, require people to undertake a major revision of their assumptions about the world; secondly, are lasting in their implications, rather than transient; and, finally, take place over a relatively short period of time so that there is little opportunity for preparation. Clearly, a victim of serious crime can be said to have experienced all of the above, which Parkes refers to collectively as a psychosocial transition (PST). Some victims of crime, then, are at risk of developing a recognised mental illness as a consequence of their experiences.

Another function of voluntary organisations is to act as *pressure groups*, attempting to promote change in large statutory bodies such as the NHS. There are long-standing groups, such as MENCAP and *ad hoc* groups which campaign for a single short-term aim, such as to save a local hospital from closure. They may be extremely effective at mobilising public opinion, which in turn puts pressure on policy makers to change their plans. In Victim Support, lobbying on relevant issues usually occurs at a national level. A recent example of successful lobbying resulted in the establishment of services at Crown Courts, with sufficient government funding to meet the objective of providing a service for all victims and other witnesses at all Crown Courts by the end of 1995. In addition, many schemes, including the national scheme, may involve themselves in promotional and awareness campaigns from time to time, resources permitting.

Many voluntary organisations have a role in *education and information*, by means of replying to letters, using the media, organising courses, or printing leaflets, newsletters and magazines. There are also telephone advice lines providing information on a wide range of topics. Some Victim Support schemes have a specialist service for victims of sexual crime, for example, and offer help lines and one-to-one support and counselling to clients. Often the clients who self-refer to this type of service are adult survivors of childhood sexual abuse who, as a result of this early trauma, have very salient mental and emotional health needs. Survivors of recent sexual crime also have quite urgent and specific physical health needs, related to pregnancy and sexually transmitted disease. Volunteers require particular skills in referral to other agencies in cases where specialist help is needed.

Other functions would include *community development*; for example, residents associations mentioned earlier, social clubs, or playgroups. Some community groups have a health promotion topic as their central focus, for example women's health groups, whilst in others health issues are covered more indirectly. Finally, groups may have a *self-help* function, and this is covered in the next chapter.

Whatever the predominant function(s) of a particular voluntary organisation, there is a central linking theme; that of *empowerment*. It has been suggested that 'There are few concepts in health promotion with as much potential as that termed "empowerment". It embodies the *raison d'être* of health promotion...' (Rissel, 1994, p. 40). What is interesting in this context is that within health promotion a concept has been embraced which has its origins firmly rooted in the social action and community psychology ideologies which are the underpinning philosophies of the modern voluntary movement (Rissel, *op. cit.*).

Rissel (*ibid*, p. 45) proposes two levels of empowerment: the psychological level, in which individuals experience greater feelings of control over their own lives, often through group membership; and the community level, in which, added to the above, there is a 'political action component in which members have actively participated'. In Victim Support it may be the volunteers and paid staff who become empowered at the community level, particularly if they have participated in lobbying campaigns, policy change and fund raising and publicity initiatives. For clients, the very focus of Victim Support is psychological empowerment. Part of the experience of being a victim of crime is the feeling of helpless rage and *disempowerment*. The volunteer has a role in supporting the client through the process which will take her or him from victim to survivor. This process involves the volunteer in active listening, acceptance and non-judgementalism, information giving and practical help where necessary. As stated earlier, the volunteer is trained to have a knowledge of the limitations of the role, and the skill to refer to a network of other agencies. In this way, Victim Support is working for health in an enabling way (Seedhouse, 1991).

Constraints to be overcome

The voluntary sector is funded in a variety of ways; in many cases voluntary organisations are core funded by the statutory agencies, although some of the larger charities rely almost solely on voluntary contributions and fund raising. An example of the latter would be the major national cancer charities, some of which operate on multi-million pound budgets. Increasingly, voluntary organisations are looking to the commercial world for funding and for resourcing in other ways.

Insecure funding for many voluntary organisations makes long-term planning difficult. Short-term funding means posts may only be offered on short-term contracts, making it difficult to attract high-calibre staff. Additionally, some small organisations have quite simple organisational structures, often relying on one key individual; this can create difficulties if the key person leaves. Clearly, problems with staffing and funding can lead to a lack of consistency and continuity.

The financing of Victim Support, as described earlier, is administered to local schemes via the national office, with core funding coming from the Home Office. Individual schemes also attract funding from their local statutory agencies, such as the police service, probation department and social services. Funders have a right to be involved, through policy and procedure, in how their resources have been used by the organisation and, at Victim Support, like many similar organisations, this is achieved by those bodies being represented on the management committee. Other members of that committee would be representatives of other community groups, staff and volunteers. Although not without their problems, management committees can be dynamic examples of collaboration in action and, whilst outside of the NHS, they might be viewed as healthy alliances in their own right (Department of Health, 1992). Many schemes also have a fund-raising committee, organising local charity events. With the police service as a potentially active partner in fund rasing, Victim Support schemes are well placed to raise money, particularly as the clients are seen as deserving. Other voluntary organisations often do not have these advantages and have to rely solely on their statutory funders. Davies and Edwards (1990) have described some of the issues faced by voluntary organisations working with statutory partners in the contract culture of the 1990s. For voluntary organisations, working to contracts can often mean quite significant shifts in practice and procedures, and some people find it problematic to try to quantify voluntary work in a business-like way, preferring to work informally. Can we ever measure tender loving care? (Perri 6 and Fieldgrass 1992, *ibid*).

There is, undoubtedly, a wide scope for health promotion in a voluntary setting. Whilst a definition of a voluntary organisation is not possible, generally the strengths include flexibility, enabling easy adaptation to exploit new opportunities, and highly-committed volunteers who, because they tend to be recruited from the locality or from the client group itself, more accurately reflect clients' concerns.

Given the plethora of voluntary organisations in the UK, about 300 000 in the narrow voluntary sector by some estimates (Perri 6 and Fieldgrass, 1992), there is a high potential for local need, specific need and highly specialised need to be met in a way that could not be met by the bureaucracy of the statutory sector. As the NHS concentrates more on mainstream activities, gaps may appear at the edges, creating an increased need for voluntary organisations. Increasingly, partnerships are being formed between the voluntary and statutory sectors, and there are numerous examples of successful collaboration between health authorities and voluntary organisations (Fieldgrass, 1992, Department of Health, 1993).

Victim Support has provided an example of the ways in which a voluntary organisation can operate in an empowering way with its clients, working within a framwork of holistic health. More directly, there is a case for Victim Support, in some of its more specialised work, to contribute to *The Health of the Nation* targets. The targets for mental health are inappropriately termed targets for *Mental Illness*. Furthermore, the main targets within this key area, as well as focusing on a disease model concentrate on suicide figures, a somewhat limiting quantification of the mental health of our nation. However, the role of voluntary agencies in this key target area, as elsewhere, is stressed in the document, and one statement, at least, would seem to relate directly to the role of an agency such as Victim Support:

> Local support for voluntary agencies, such as those that support people at high risk for depression, should be improved in order to strengthen the role that they play. (Department of Health, *ibid*, p. 89).

Perhaps the time has come for the statutory mental health services to become active partners of victim support schemes. This would be an interesting development for an organisation which has traditionally been perceived in connection with the various areas of the criminal justice system.

It is clear from the preceding analysis that voluntary organisations play a crucial role in our nation's health. Such is the diversity of the sector, however, that no one organisation could be said to be typical. Nevertheless, the example of Victim Support has illustrated some of the potentials and constraints for health promotion in a voluntary setting.

References

Davies, A. & Edwards, K. (1990). *Twelve Charity Contracts*. Directory of Social Change.
Department of Health (1992). *The Health of the Nation*. London: HMSO.
Department of Health (1993). *Working Together for Better Health*. London: HMSO.
Downie, R.S., Fyfe, C., & Tannahill, A. (1992). *Health Promotion: Models and Values*. Oxford: Oxford University Press.
Fieldgrass, J. (1992). *Partnerships in Health Promotion*. London: Health Education Authority.
Kenner, C. (1986). *Whose Needs Count?* London: National Council for Voluntary Organisations NCVO Publications.
Knight, B. (1993). *Voluntary Action*. London: Centris.
Murray-Parkes, C. (1993). Bereavement as a psychosocial transition: process of adaptation to change. In M. S. Stroebe, W. Stroebe & R. O. Hansson *Handbook of Bereavement*. Cambridge:Cambridge University Press.
National Association of Victim Support (1989). *Annual Report*. London: NAVS.
Perri 6 (1991). *What is a Voluntary Organisation? Defining the Voluntary and Non-Profit Sectors*. London: National Council for Voluntary Organisations/ NCVO Publications.
Perri 6 & Fieldgrass, J. (1992). *Snapshots of the Voluntary Sector Today*. London: National Council For Voluntary Organisations/NCVO Publications.
Priority Focus (1994). *What Would Improve Your Health, Happiness and Well Being?* A survey of the health needs of residents of Swindon. Report to Healthy Thamesdown Working Party. Sheffield: Priority Focus.
Rissel, C. (1994). Empowerment: the holy grail of health promotion? In *Health Promotion International*, 9(1).
Seedhouse, D. (1994). *Fortress NHS*. Chichester: John Wiley & Sons.
Seedhouse, D. (1991). *Health: The Foundations for Achievement*. Chichester: John Wiley.

17 *A self-help approach to health promotion*

Jan Myers and Kate Marsden

Over the past decade there has been a proliferation of self-help groups in Britain. This follows closely the American trend for a diversity of groups based on individual needs around health and social welfare issues. These self-help or mutual-aid organisations can serve any number of purposes depending on the make-up of the members, but generally groups consist of people 'who share the same concern or life experience' (Jezewski, 1986, p. 5). They can also include people indirectly affected by the issue, such as friends, carers and relatives. Most importantly, groups and their activities are managed and controlled by their members.

This development and sharing of experiential knowledge can lead to the empowerment of individual group members. As Mullender and Ward (1991, p. 12) explain:

> ... in groups personal troubles can be translated into common concerns. The demoralising isolation of private misfortune ... can be placed in the course of collective enterprise with a new sense of self confidence and potency, as well as tangible practical gains which individuals on their own could not contemplate.

However, mutual aid begins with 'the desire to take oneself in hand' (St Amand and Clavette, 1992, p. 18). In this way, in order to become a member of a self-help group, an individual must own (or own up to) an issue and therefore must be conducive to, or seeking, change. For example, persons who join Alcoholics Anonymous do so in the knowledge that they are alcoholic and want to do something about it. Hatch and Hinton (cited in the Community Project Foundation's *Action For Health*, 1988) stated that there was both room, and a need, for people to be able to define their problems and their own forms of support. If we take Thorogood's suggestion in Bunton and MacDonald (1992, pp. 77–80) that health promotion should 'start where people are developmentally ... start where people are emotionally ... start where people are socially', then self-help groups provide a good thermometer to all three areas.

The connection between self-help and health promotion

In this way, there is a valid connection between health promotion and self-help, where health promotion is concerned with providing opportunities for people to take decisions that are conducive to a healthy lifestyle. Within this, health promotion enables people to work increasingly to a greater understanding of health issues and, in seeking to 'improve or protect health through behavioural, biological, socio-economic and environmental changes' (Gann, 1986, p. 12), it closely allies itself with the philosophy of self-help. Both are concerned with a holistic picture of the person. This wide approach to health promotion is defined by the World Health Organisation quoted in Fieldgrass (1992, p. 7), where health promotion is seen as a 'unifying concept for those who recognise the need for change in the ways and conditions of living, in order to promote health.' A key element of this is 'supporting the principle of self-help and self-care movements, to allow people to form their own directions for managing the health of their own community' (*ibid*, 1992, p. 8). This, then, provides a guide to an essential and effective linking between health professionals and self-help groups.

Self-help groups provide many opportunities for helping one another in promoting health, whether this is within groups or externally working alongside health professionals. Groups may not only educate their members in disease management but also about the health care system and the way it works. Toffler (1981, p. 25) has looked at the rapid growth of self-help and with it the basic shift in roles of what he terms *prosumers*, that is people relying on themselves for things for which they have previously depended on others. This can be demonstrated in many groups dealing with chronic illness; for example, self management of diabetes. With this is the confluent change of the professional from expert to 'listener, teacher and guide who works with the patient or client' (Toffler, 1981. p. 279). A key part of this shift is to value the knowledge gained by self-help group members from their day-to-day experience of living, for example with HIV, with chronic illness, or with life after a heart attack.

This growth of knowledge and sharing of experiences of self-help group members is seen as a central part of the helping process within groups. One allergy and behavioural support group illustrated in Baker (1987, pp. 5–6) found that each member *became an expert* in their own field, and that a consequence of this was increased confidence of group members. Furthermore, membership of a 'well supported group increases take up of statutory services by sufferers' (Action for Health, 1988, p. 41). Part of this may also include more appropriate use of statutory services because groups are providing a major part of the emotional and psychological support for individuals. Louis Medvene of the California Self-Help Centre has compiled selected highlights of research on the effectiveness of self-help groups, several of which show a lower crisis admission into hospital or showed a better understanding of coping with illness; higher self-esteem, fewer feelings of shame, a more positive outlook and in some cases a better patient–doctor relationship. It would seem, then, that self-help groups can be a way of fostering mutual understanding between health professionals and individual patients, and of improving communication. It therefore places self-help in an important position within primary care which in turn can be supported and nurtured by health promotion specialists, and where the symbiotic nature of this relationship can perhaps be acknowledged.

In order to look at why this relationship needs to be enhanced, we have to look at the complementary nature of self-help to professional care and its effect on health. A member of a group for depressives in Canada believed that self-help helped her to retain her health: 'It's good for my mental health. I get a lot out of listening to others' (St Armand and Clavette, 1992, p. 71) and again, 'I for one would be much more open with a person who is like me than a professional' (*ibid*, p. 97). Another was even more emphatic: 'I haven't had a depression since we started Depressives Anonymous' (*ibid*, p. 121). A mental health group in Sheffield also emphasised the health promotion aspects of the group, not because they talked about their illnesses all the time but that the group gave companionship and a comfortable environment to talk over practical problems. This group started as a way of administering bus passes to people with mental health problems, but increasingly found that its drop-in resource helped people to find their feet when they came out of hospital when they were *feeling lost*.

Where resources like the drop-in centre are run by groups, it is important for professionals to use the resources appropriately. Groups can often find themselves overwhelmed by individuals being referred by professionals when more structured, supervised support may be needed. Individuals need to self-refer; that is, they need to be able to make a choice whether to go to a group or not. Professionals can aid this process by giving information to allow the individual to make an informed choice; what Wilson (1994) refers to as 'putting people in touch'.

Some groups work closely with health professionals, often with the expressed intent of promoting health among members. The Cardiac Support Group in Nottingham actively promotes health at its monthly meetings by inviting a wide range of speakers ranging from cardiac specialists, paramedics, physiotherapists and pharmacists, to social welfare professionals who can advise on employment, benefits and aids. Here, the health professionals take an active role in supporting the group by attending meetings when asked by the members. The running and, therefore, control and management of the group falls squarely on the shoulders of the members. The Positive Health Group in Nottingham finds that links with professionals help to create a better understanding of health but also of the way health agencies work. The group has a more generalist approach to health and again invites speakers on a wide range of subjects. Here, the rationale is that group members may at some point in their lives be affected by, for example, a stroke, dementia or osteoporosis. In this way, there is a raising of awareness, a more positive approach to 'growing old' and also an active way of providing space to relax and learn. This also raises confidence in the health service, an important issue in health promotion. Loss of faith in a general practitioner, a hospital or nursing staff may have a detrimental effect on the individual. As the name of the group implies it is a positive way of looking at both health and illness.

Some groups actually take on board active health promotion and encourage service providers. One such group in Nottingham, OSCAR, is concerned with sickle cell anaemia. Working closely with a health centre, OSCAR was instrumental in the setting up and supporting of a sickle cell and thalassaemia project sited within the centre. Another example is in the area of gay sexual health where self-help has been an integral part in health provision; being seen by one health promotion officer as providing a collective and empowered response to HIV where statutory services had not responded or perhaps not even recognised a need. This long tradition of self-help in the gay community could partly be seen as a response to being a disenfranchised part of society in relation to health care and other service provision. Likewise, groups may set up where traditional medicine has proven ineffective or, as in the case of Tranquilliser Withdrawal Groups, because of it. Yet they can still be seen as adhering to a health promotion role.

Wilson (1994, forthcoming) in her research on good practice between self-help groups and professionals, looked at how groups identify themselves; relationships between groups and professionals and the ways in which professionals can support and develop self-help. Groups fall into three categories, those working within the health system, those working alongside the system and yet others who identify themselves as independent. Where groups are independent they may still recognise the importance of dialogue with purchasers and providers of health services, if only to get across their own point of view. A fourth category would be the Fellowship groups such as Alcoholics Anonymous and Overeaters Anonymous where autonomy is a major principle and so precludes any liaison with organisations outside the fellowship.

Of the groups interviewed, Wilson found that many welcomed informal opportunities to influence how services are provided. Again, many groups have felt overwhelmed by the burden of the consultation process. Wilson found that few saw it as a major part of their role and that professionals needed to be 'aware of the risks of diverting a group from their original aims or commandeering their limited time and energy' (Wilson, 1994).

The relationships between statutory services and self-help

How health professionals support self-help initiatives can affect the success or failure of a group. This can be a simple act of support such as displaying a poster advertising a group, an acknowledgement that the group exists and a willingness to put people in touch with the group. On the other end of the scale it may be help with material or monetary resources, access to meeting rooms, or support and training for group members to enhance their skills for running a group. In addition, it may be to provide assistance to groups to evaluate their work or to help in times of crisis. Health promoters can also act as a signpost to other services when professional back-up is needed. This is also highlighted by Wilson's research. She found many ways in which professionals could help groups. The strength of this help was that it was 'sensitive background support, based on community work, enabling principles and offered over a long period' (*ibid*, 1994).

Some professionals may need to change practices or their perceptions of the needs of their patients, and this is also a role that health promoters may explore further. In one instance, two health service professionals stated that as 'a result of running short courses for a depression and anxiety group and observing the progress the group had made, they are considering rethinking their own practice in order to look at ways in which it might become more user-centred' (Abraham and Webb, 1989, p. 33).

The responses of health professionals to self-help groups have been changing over the years, which also dovetails with the outreach work being done by health promotion officers. If, as Ashton and Seymour (1988) suggest, health promotion works through effective community action by education for health, providing information and developing skills, then, sourcing and resourcing self-help groups is a way of reaching a wider community and providing greater equality of opportunity in relation to access to information and resources. One health promotion officer in Nottingham believes strongly in the interconnection of self-help and health promotion, understanding that this relationship is a two-way process offering mutual benefits to both group and professional. This understanding can then be drawn upon to provide concrete ways of working: this particular health promotion team works closely with a Bangladeshi group – here, the group members set the agenda and the health promotion workers provide the relevant information. Similarly, Wilson (1994) found that alliances worked best where there was this kind of reciprocity.

Moreover, in a changing health care system, with greater recognition of the patient's voice, market forces, quality standard setting and outcomes, self-help groups are becoming increasingly recognised as a valuable source of consumer feedback. The result is seen in concentrated efforts to include self-help groups in multifarious consultation exercises. Indeed, the Society of Health Promotion Officers has indicators of good practice in relation to services offered which are embodied in the *Health for All 2000*, and which include community participation and the role of advocacy and empowerment (Fieldgrass, 1992, p. 23). This ties in with Wilson's suggestion of an approach which makes effective but appropriate use of group members' knowledge and experience, to develop good working relationships based on standardised good practice which includes a demystification of the provision of services and a subsequent lessening in the use of organisational jargon. Perhaps, again, a lesson can be learned from why people join self-help groups which, in turn, can help to make this a more positive experience for all involved: 'Dr X will tell him things that he doesn't understand, and I'll explain it in simpler words. This is a critical thing, explaining it in simple terms instead of big fancy words' (St Amand and Clavette, 1992, p. 111). It is also in this arena that health promotion officers have a role to play, not only as health educators to the community but in their role as trainers for a wide range of health professionals.

One of the general principles of the Strategic Plan 1990–1995 states that the Health Education Authority wants to 'work in partnership with other organisations and with individuals' (Health Education Authority, 1989, p. 5) and that 'the voluntary sector also has considerable potential for health education through its links with local communities and groups, its support for self help and advocacy of wider health policies' (*ibid*, 1989, p. 16). If this is the case, then perhaps it must also look at how it puts this into practice. *Partnership* implies an equality of relationship which does not currently exist, but which can be explored by health promoters through the way information is published and distributed, support is given and agendas are set. Perhaps *active alliances* would be a better description of where professionals and self-help groups are working well together.

These active alliances provide a real pay-off in terms of patient care and professional time and should not be seen as Hadley (1988, p. 98) points out as 'inadmissible evidence of ... professional failure'. Moreover, if health promotion is seen, as can be suggested, as geared by the more short-term, specific targets of *The Health of the Nation*, then issues which underlie the promotion of healthy lifestyles such as raised self-esteem or assertiveness – all the positive aspects pointed to by self-help group members time and again – are seen as being at the soft end of the quality circle. The constraints of this are that the very work which promotes this enabling, empowering role is then seen to be peripheral. It would be a shame to think that the bridge between the professional and self-help world, possibly provided by health promotion in a positive and real way, could be eroded in a backlash to community development approaches. Furthermore, that contact between the two sectors could become strained as groups start up in response to perceived gaps in services as they see an NHS becoming more privatised.

However, the converse of this is, as Bunton and MacDonald (1992, p. 6) point out, that 'the knowledge base of health promotion would appear to be growing more multi-disciplinary, as the professional background of health promoters is becoming more varied' and therefore this may open up opportunities for a variety of methodological approaches to health promotion, including working with groups. Many of the professionals interviewed by Wilson (1994) had received little or no training in group-work techniques. It remains the case that good working relationships between groups and health professionals are inconsistent, relying on individual interest rather than a system of good practice. Health promotion officers are well placed to raise the profile of self-help with a growing number of actors on the health promotion stage: general practitioners, pharmacists and hospitals. However, in order to do so they also need to familiarise themselves with the growing phenomenon of self-help.

It may be that health promotion officers can and should actively seek out groups to offer their support (at the same time understanding that it will be a group's decision whether or not to accept such help). As this increasing collaboration brings the two sides closer together, care must be taken that the professional world does not overtake the self-help world completely (Wilson, forthcoming). As Abraham and Webb (1989, p. 30) emphasise, self-help should not be incorporated into the statutory sector, for to do so 'would lose many of its most valued features, for example its independence and autonomy – and must therefore stay outside in order to offer an alternative to formal organised and bureaucratic health structure'.

References

Abraham, F. & Webb, B. (1989). *Mental Health and Self Help Support.* London: Tavistock Institute of Human Relations.

Anderson, A. (1991). The Victoria experience in health promotion and health information in a city centre. *Health Libraries Review.* 8(1), 33–34.

Ashton, J. & Seymour, H. (1988). *The New Public Health.* Milton Keynes: Open University Press.

Baker, J. (1987). *Self Help Groups and Professional Agencies: Improving Understanding and Co-operation.* Hull:Department of Social Policy and Professional Studies.

Billingham, K. (1990). *Learning Together: A Health Resource Pack for Working with Groups.* Nottingham: Nottingham Community Health.

Bolton, M. (1991). Health of the nation: where do voluntary organisations fit in to government plans to improve health promotion. *NCVO News* (November), 6.

Bornat, J., Phillipson, C. & Ward, S. (1985). *Manifesto for Old Age.* London:-Pluto.

Bradburn, J., Maher, E. J., Young, J. & Young, T. (1992). Community based support groups: an undervalued resource? *Clinical Oncology, 4,* 377–380.

Bunton, R. & MacDonald, G. (1992). Health promotion discipline or disciplines. In R. Bunton & G. MacDonald (eds), *Health Promotion: Disciplines and Diversity.* London/New York: Routledge.

Community Project Foundation (1988). *Action For Health: Initiatives in Local Communities.* London: Community Project Foundation.

Durand, Y. (1990). Cultural sensitivity in practice. In C. Chris & M Pearl (eds), *Women AIDS and Activism.* New York: Southend Press.

Ewles, L. & Simnett, I. (1991). *Promoting Health: A Practical Guide to Health Information.* 2nd edn. London: Wiley.

Fieldgrass, J. (1992). *Partnerships in Health: Collaboration between the Statutory and Voluntary Sectors.* London: Health Education Authority.

Gann, R. (1986). *The Health Information Handbook.* London: Gower.

Hadley, J. (1988). A Fashionable Minefield. *Health Service Journal, 98*(5103), 620–621.

Harrison, D. & Ashcroft, A. (1994). Early warning systems. *The Health Service Journal* (6 October), 38–30.

Health Promotion Research Trust (1989). *Annual Report.* Cambridge: HPRT.

Health Promotion Service (1993–1994). *Annual Review.* Nottingham Community Health: NHS Trust.

Jezewski, T. (1986). *Getting Better Known Self Help Groups,* 2nd edn. Cottesloe, Australia: Western Institute of Self Help.

Katz, A. H. (1987). *Partners in Wellness: Self Help Groups and Professionals.* California: Department of Mental Health Office of Prevention.

Medvene, L. J. (received by Self Help Team 1992). *Selected Highlights of Research on Effectiveness of Self Help Groups.* California: Self Help Center UCLA.

Mullender, A. & Ward, D. (1991). *Self Directed Groupwork.* London: Whiting & Birch.

St Amand, N. & Clavette, H. (1992). *Self Help and Mental Health: Beyond Psychiatry.* Canada: Canadian Council on Social Development.

Thorogood, N. (1992). What is the relevance of sociology for health promotion? In R.Bunton & G.MacDonald, *Health Promotion: Disciplines and Diversity.* London/New York: Routledge.

Toffler, A. (1981). *The Third Wave.* London: Pan.

White, B. J. & Madara, E. J. (1992). *The Self Help Source Book: Finding and Forming Mutual Aid Self Help Groups,* 4th edn. New Jersey:American Self Help Clearing House.

Wilson, J. (1994). *Social Care Research 60: Self Help Groups and Professionals*. York: Joseph Rowntree Foundation.

Wilson, J. (forthcoming). *Two Worlds: Self Help Groups and Professionals*. Birmingham: Venture.

Wilson, J. (forthcoming). *Valuing Self Help: Guidelines for Professionals in Working with Self Help Goups*. London: Arena.

SECTION SIX

Workplace

18 Overview of health promotion in the workplace

Diana Sanders and Sally Crowe

The importance of health promotion in the workplace is increasingly being recognised, not only to prevent disease, disability or death caused by hazards at work and the working environment, but also because the workplace provides a setting and the opportunity to tackle health issues and improve the health of employees (Schilling, 1989; Health Education Authority, 1992 a,b,c; Trent Regional Health Authority, 1993). National policies such as *The Health of the Nation*, 'Health at Work in the NHS' and Health and Safety legislation endorse and encourage workplace health initiatives. Several national human resource initiatives such as 'Investors in People' contribute to a coordinated planned approach and can enhance health promotion initiatives. Health promotion interventions in the workplace are becoming increasingly common, particularly in larger organisations. The increase in activity has evolved due to a variety of factors: recognition of the costs of employee ill-health; response to internal and external pressures to be seen as caring employers; and health and safety and European legislation. However, as will be discussed in this chapter, the UK lags behind other countries in both the extent of provision of programmes and in evaluating such programmes. Therefore, drawing conclusions about the benefits of health promotion in the workplace, and making recommendations as to effective programmes, is limited. This chapter provides an overview of the extent of health promotion in the workplace, looking at the literature from North America and Europe as well as the UK, with case studies illustrating effective programmes in general health promotion and in ways of tackling two main areas of concern: smoking and stress. The chapter concludes with recommendations about the characteristics of successful health promotion programmes at work. The chapter is based on a review of the literature on workplace health promotion (Sanders, 1993).

The extent of health promotion in the workplace

Surveys of public and private-sector employers and trade unions in the UK have shown that health promotion programmes are receiving increasing attention, although they are by no means universal (Webb *et al.*, 1988; Watson, 1992). In 1991, the extent and nature of employee health and welfare programmes in private and public-sector organisations was surveyed (Watson, 1992). A postal questionnaire to 300 organisations, with a 50 per cent response rate, and interviews with 12 respondents revealed that around half of respondents had provided health promotion programmes, with higher rates of provision in private sector and health authorities compared to local authorities. More recently, the Heath Education Authority surveyed a sample of 1344 workplaces in England, using telephone interviews, to obtain an accurate picture of workplace health activity (Health Education Authority, 1993). Workplace health promotion was seen to be a very important issue by 69 per cent of very large organisations but by only 41 per cent of small workplaces. Overall, 40 per cent of all workplaces undertook at least one major health-related activity in the previous year, and the likelihood of having at least one major programme increased with workplace size. Smoking was considered the most important health-related activity. Eighty-one per cent of large companies with more than 500 employees had smoking-related activities; however, only 31 per cent of small companies had attempted to tackle the problem of smoking in the workplace.

Overall, these findings are moderately encouraging, but must be interpreted with caution. The degree of reported health promotion activity may be an overestimate due to response bias: companies who have an interest in health promotion may be more likely to respond to surveys than those with little interest and little or no activity, giving a much lower rate of health promotion in the UK workplace. Philo *et al.* (1992), reviewing the literature on the extent of workplace health promotion in the UK, conclude that, compared with other countries, there is a very low rate of workplace health initiatives. There is no legal requirement for occupational health services except in exceptionally dangerous occupations, and little development of a coordinated occupational health service in the NHS (Harvey, 1988; Philo *et al.*, 1992). Health promotion programmes have tended to be adopted on an *ad hoc* basis rather than as a specific policy for health promotion, with very little systematic evaluation of the effectiveness of programmes (Webb *et al.*, 1988).

The benefits of health promotion programmes

Workplace health promotion is well established in the US and Canada, and many initiatives have been shown to yield benefits which justify the costs (Eriksen, 1988; Warner *et al.*, 1988; Ashton, 1989; Pencack, 1991; Bovell, 1992). In the UK, Bovell suggests that although there is too little evidence that proves conclusively that workplace health promotion leads to financial benefits for employers and health gains for staff, there are benefits in a number of areas that need considering.

- *Absences from work* The evidence suggests those workplace health promotion interventions that are systematically organised, available to all staff, well resourced, supported by management and continue for some time, lead to significant reductions in the overall level of absenteeism. Falls in absenteeism of between 9 and 29 per cent have been reported, with an increase in absence rates in control groups not subject to the health promotion intervention.
- *Productivity* Research indicates that health promotion in the workplace can lead to a 4 per cent gain in productivity.
- *Staff attitude and morale* Health promotion programmes are associated with improvements in morale, assessed by measures such as attitudes towards the organisation and staff relations.
- *Staff Turnover* Turnover is reduced following the introduction of health promotion programmes.

Although clear benefits arising from workplace health promotion have been demonstrated in North America, the extrapolation to the UK workplace may be limited, given that the main incentive for these initiatives in North America is to reduce employer-borne health insurance costs, whereas the motivation in the UK may not be so clear (Ashton, 1989). As UK employers increasingly offer private health insurance schemes to a wide range of employees, the economic benefits of workplace health promotion programmes experienced in North America become more relevant to the UK. Extrapolation of the effects on productivity and absenteeism from America to the UK may be more reasonable: although North American workplace initiatives may have been started to reduce health-care costs to employers, most of the benefits are seen in areas other than medical care expenditure, such as reduced absenteeism, improved productivity, morale and company image. Bovell (1992) believes that if UK programmes were tailored to the different circumstances of the employees and organisations as in American programmes, there is no reason to believe these would not yield comparably positive results.

Although many health promotion programmes are in progress in the UK, and many organisations believe that their health promotion and screening programmes are returning economic benefits, much of the information is unpublished and many programmes have not been formally evaluated. In many cases there is little incentive for an organisation to invest time and money on formal studies. Even though a large number of organisations expect to see a fall in absenteeism as a result of their workplace health promotion activities, only a quarter have tried to measure changes in absenteeism in any systematic way, but these companies do report lower absence levels, indicating it may be a tangible benefit of health promotion in the workplace (Industrial Relations Service, 1989a).

Who benefits from health promotion in the workplace?

Two of the challenges confronting workplace health promotion programmes are firstly, ensuring that programmes are accessible to all sectors of the workforce, and secondly, maintaining participation in the programmes. In many health promotion and screening programmes, uptake is lower in those who have higher risk factors, such as smoking, or whose health status is already compromised due to socioeconomic disadvantages. In the US, participation rates in workplace programmes vary from 20–40 per cent for on-site programmes and 10–25 per cent for programmes outside the workplace (Lovato and Green, 1990). Most programmes have drop-out rates of between 30 and 70 per cent in the first three to six months. There is evidence that employees at higher risk for cardiovascular disease participate less in health promotion programmes (Rost, 1990; Lovato and Green, 1990): participants tend to be non-smokers, more concerned about their health, more knowledgeable about health issues, more educated, younger in age, using fewer health services, and with lower absenteeism and turnover rates (Lovato and Green, 1990; Alexy, 1991). Barriers to participation in health promotion programmes included shift work, working overtime, responsibilities at home, and distance from work (Alexy, 1991). No similar body of data on participation and maintenance is available for the UK. One study of cancer education programmes (Health Education Authority, 1991a) indicates that male blue-collar workers are likely to be reluctant to attend cancer education activities. Several recommendations for improving participation rates have been described by Bovell (1992) and Philo *et al.* (1992), including surveys to assess and target individual needs and increase employees' involvement in programme development and evaluation by improving the process of consultation, collaboration and participation across all staff groups. Careful pre-programme individual assessments to identify and address environmental and individual factors that may cause an individual to drop out may also improve participation (Lovato and Green, 1990).

Health promotion programmes at work

Some examples of workplace health promotion programmes are given below, followed by case studies of initiatives to tackle two major health problems, smoking and stress. Other examples are cited in Sanders (1993).

General programmes

Case Study: Polaroid UK (Ashton 1989; Matheson 1987; Industrial Relations Service 1989b; Anon 1990)
Polaroid (UK) is part of a US-based multinational company, with a British manufacturing plant located near Dumbarton, Scotland. The 'Vale of Leven Health Promotion Project' started in 1986 for its 1400 employees. The first phase focused on improving employees lifestyles and screening for coronary heart disease (CHD) risk factors. Employees were given the opportunity to contribute to the debate on the precise form of health promotion package offered, through elected Employee Advisory Groups. A Smoking Policy was developed and introduced and 'Quit' groups were offered to help individuals stop smoking.

Evaluation Many of the employees found to have risk factors for CHD were able to reduce them: for example, of the 555 men initially screened, 24 per cent had a cholesterol level of more than 6.5 mm/l; at second screening one month later, the figure had reduced to 10 per cent. Of 646 women screened, the 15 per cent above the criterion had also been reduced to 9 per cent by the second test. The mean fall in cholesterol was 1.3 micro moles for men, 0.7 for women. The reduction in blood cholesterol levels following dietary advice was particularly marked in men aged 40–49, of whom the 30 per cent above the criterion before intervention was reduced to 13 per cent after. The measuring of cholesterol levels and feeding back results to individuals was felt to be an essential part of the programme. 'Quit' groups were not successful in helping any smokers to stop. Absenteeism rates fell from 6.3 per cent in 1982 to 3.7 per cent in October 1989. The company estimates that the reduction in absenteeism has saved the company around £113 000 per year.

Case Study: The Welsh Heart Programme (Clarkson *et al.*, 1991)
'Heartbeat Wales' was set up in 1985 to test the feasibility and effectiveness of a national prevention programme for cardiovascular disease. The programme identified the workplace as a key setting for health promotion. The components introduced for smoking included educational programmes for new employees, Look After Yourself (LAY) classes, extension of occupational health services to cover counselling and health appraisal, and smoking policy development. For psychosocial health, self-help groups and LAY classes were introduced. The key steps in the development of workplace programmes

included agenda setting and awareness-raising discussion conferences and seminars, aimed at the various parties with roles in health at work; development of support materials; specific projects such as the Heartbeat Award Scheme for catering establishments, Make Health your Business Award, Well Welsh, a health screening programme for commerce and industry, and LAY.

Evaluation This focused on the extent of provision of programmes, rather than outcome or effectiveness. The programme was evaluated in 1989; a telephone survey was conducted of over 200 private companies with more than 100 employees. Results indicated that interest in health issues is steadily growing, with 27 per cent of companies reporting a smoking policy, although policies on stress were rare (4 per cent). More than half of the companies reported that they offered health screening services for staff, and 38 per cent of companies offered staff counselling services. No information was available on the uptake or effectiveness of programmes.

Smoking and the workplace

Smoking ranks alongside some of the major occupational hazards as a priority for action by employers, trade unions and health promotion organisations (Webb *et al.*, 1988). The workplace has many advantages as a location for smoking-cessation interventions. Large populations of smokers can be contacted, offered programmes and followed up, and workplace programmes are likely to be accessible to smokers, particularly if offered on-site and during working hours (Hallett, 1986). There is enormous potential to reduce the risks to both smokers and non-smokers, of secondary smoking in the workplace (Department of Health and Social Security, 1988).

There are two approaches to smoking in the workplace (Hallett, 1986); smoking policies and interventions to help individuals to stop smoking. Policies to limit smoking in the workplace are becoming increasingly common, in both public and private sectors (Jenkins *et al.*, 1987; Batten, 1988, 1990; Industrial Relations Service, 1992a,b; Department of Health, 1992; Hurst, 1992; Health Education Authority, 1993). Most of the evidence for the effectiveness of workplace smoking-cessation initiatives comes from the US (reviewed by Sanders 1993). Overall, whilst many companies and employers express interest in smoking policies, mainly in response to health and safety legislation and concerns about passive smoking and economic factors, their development remains patchy, and there is a gap between development and implementation. It is not known whether workplace policies affect smoking prevalence directly, but social acceptability and desirability of smoking may be influenced by such restrictions, as well as protecting individuals from passive smoking.

Case Study: Smoking in Spanish hospitals (Batlle et al., 1991)

The problem of smoking is far more severe in Spanish hospitals than in the UK: 62 per cent of the general working population, and 35 per cent of doctors smoke. Around a third smoke in front of their patients, half allow patients to smoke in waiting rooms, and a third never advise their patients to stop smoking. A comprehensive smoking policy was introduced in a hospital near Barcelona, with the aims of reducing tobacco consumption amongst hospital staff and creating an awareness amongst staff of their exemplary role as health professionals. The policy included a number of different activities: workshops on the consequences of smoking; smoking restrictions in hospital; and help for smokers who wished to stop smoking, using group therapy and nicotine gum. A key factor was the involvement of hospital staff in each stage of the programme; as a result, the majority of staff felt positive and supportive of the programme. To evaluate the intervention, a survey of smoking habits and attitudes amongst hospital staff was conducted before the programme and two and a half years after its implementation. At baseline, 51 per cent of staff smoked. After three years, the rate of smoking had fallen to 40 per cent of workers, with physicians and nurses being the most likely to have stopped smoking. There was also a significant positive change in attitudes amongst health professionals, particularly in their views of advising patients to stop smoking, and in creating smoke-free waiting rooms.

The results of this case study show that a well-motivated planning group and a well thought out health promotion strategy, actively involving staff, adapted to the specific situation and conditions of the hospital, and with the explicit support of health administration and health authority, can lead to the implementation of an effective, comprehensive smoking policy, even in a situation that appears far more difficult than the situation in the UK health service. The more effective smoking policies in the UK, noted by Webb *et al.* (1988), similarly emphasise the cooperation and involvement of employees.

Stress and the workplace

Managing stress is increasingly seen as a priority for both employees and employers. In a survey of 40 large organisations representing employers and unions, stress was given a high priority as a cause of ill-health (Webb *et al.*, 1988). Stress has been linked to many different aspects of ill-health and lack of well-being. Work and the way it is organised can directly or indirectly give rise to stress (DeFrank and Cooper, 1987; Cooper and Payne, 1988; Jee and Reason, 1988; Klimes, 1989; Health Education Authority, 1988, 1990; Jenkins and Coney, 1992; National Association of Staff Support, 1992; Creed, 1993; Owen, 1993). The costs of stress to the individual are potentially enormous. In addition, the total cost of stress to British industry is thought to be vast. At least 80 million working days are lost each year due to ailments associated with or exacerbated by stress, costing employers £3.7 billion per annum. Drink-related absenteeism related to stress is estimated to cost industry around £700 million per year; sickness absence due to hangovers accounts for between 8 and 14 million lost working days per year. It has been shown that people with high job strain have significantly higher absence rates, and that there is a clear association between sickness absence and perceived health (National Association for Staff Support, 1992). In the USA, employers are increasingly being held liable for the health problems of their employees that result from job stress, and in the last 10 years, work-related stress has become a leading cause of worker's compensation claims (Jee and Reason, 1988). In the UK, a small number of cases are in progress of employees suing their employers for psychological stress at work: should these cases be successful, they will no doubt set a precedent for future legal action.

There are two main approaches to dealing with stress at work (Payne and Firth-Cozens, 1987; Murphy, 1988; Arroba and James, 1990). One is to view the individual as being unable to cope with work demands or pressures from outside the workplace, and offer stress or anxiety management courses or counselling and training in management skills. The aim of this approach is to either increase the individual's resistance to the harmful effects of stress, or to increase their ability to cope with it. Whilst the approach may have a preventive component and may help individuals in the short term, it treats symptoms and not the causes of stress. The second approach is to change the working environment and tackle the causes of stress in the work setting, involving changes in policies and practices and staff at all levels of the organisation.

Individual interventions to manage stress at work are by far the most common (Klimes, 1989; National Association for Staff Support, 1992; Owen, 1993), with most attention given to Stress Management Training and workplace counselling programmes (Sanders, 1993). The following case study illustrates an example of a staff counselling service.

Case Study: Counselling in the Post Office (Allinson *et al.*, 1989; Cooper and Sadri, 1991)
The Post Office, one of the largest employers in the UK, recognised

in the early 1980s that there was a need to provide some form of emotional and psychological support to employees. The Counselling Pilot Study included several components: provision of an open-access specialist counselling resource with individual counselling; a training programme for occupational health professionals to enhance first-line counselling skills; and a stress education seminar programme to train occupational health doctors and nurses to educate line managers in the identification and management of stress. Within the first three years, a major cluster of counselling had been on mental health issues, mainly anxiety and depression, forming 46 per cent of the caseload. Other issues brought to the service included relationship problems, alcohol problems, bereavement, assault, physical illness or disability and social problems. Two hundred and fifty employees attending the counselling service and a control group consisting of a comparable group of 100 postal employees took part in the study. The effectiveness and benefits of the service from the individual client's viewpoint was assessed by comparing psychological test measurements of well-being and attitudes of clients with a matched control group. After counselling, the client group showed improvements in all areas of psychological well-being and behaviour. There was a decline in clinical anxiety levels, somatic anxiety, depression and an increase in self-esteem. The client group showed reduced dependence on alcohol, coffee and smoking as coping mechanisms, and greater use of exercise and relaxation techniques. At the organisational level, objective measurements of sickness absence were used. Prior to counselling, the client group had an average absence level of 32.5 days in a six-month period; this fell to 11.1 days, a significant reduction. No changes during a comparable period were found in the control group. There were no changes, however, in job satisfaction and organisational commitment. Overall, the Post Office was able to demonstrate that there are definite cost and organisational benefits from the introduction of a counselling service and that the benefits outweigh the costs.

Presently, interventions aimed at the individual are by far the most prevalent form of initiative. Whilst stress management training may have a limited role in addressing stress, and occupational counselling schemes have been shown to be effective, there is a flavour of victim blaming, and they offer only a limited solution to the problem of stress at work. Organisational change has an important role in not only reducing but also preventing stress at work. Unfortunately, very few examples of good practice, let alone those which have been evaluated, are available. One exception is North Derbyshire Health Authority, which established a working group on staff stress in 1986. The working group has conducted a survey of staff stress, prepared a strategy for coping with stress, strengthened the counselling service for staff, supported stress awareness and management workshops, and collaborated in research evaluating 'innovation' as a method of coping with stress (Bunce and West 1993). It is likely that a combination of approaches will prove to be the most effective in tackling stress at work.

Characteristics of successful health promotion programmes in the workplace

Despite the lack of research and evaluation in the area, it is possible to draw some conclusions about what contributes to effective health promotion programmes at work. For general health promotion programmes, as well as the specific topic areas of smoking and stress, the following principles contribute to successful programme implementation and outcome (Sanders, 1993):

1. The most effective programmes are those with a coordinated and planned approach.
2. Staff at all levels of the organisation, both management and employees, as well as unions, should be involved in planning, implementing and evaluating programmes.
3. The programmes should have backing from senior management and be seen to be taken seriously by the organisation.
4. Programmes should be directly related to the expressed and measured needs of the workforce.
5. A range of health promotion interventions should be offered.
6. The effects of health promotion campaigns may reduce over time; therefore sustaining campaigns over a long period is important.
7. The most effective programmes involve personal, face-to-face and individualised health promotion activities, rather than general educational programmes. This is particularly the case for the two topic areas, smoking and stress.
8. There is some evidence from the literature that it is more effective to target high-risk groups rather than only offer general health promotion programmes.

Compared to other countries, there is a low rate of workplace health promotion initiatives in the UK. There is at present no legal requirement for occupational health services and little development of a coordinated occupational health service in the NHS. Most programmes emphasise individual behaviour and lifestyle issues rather than organisational and environmental factors. However, as discussed in this chapter, the benefits of health promotion at work are well established in the US and Canada, and reviews of the literature demonstrate that health promotion programmes in the workplace can lead to a significant decrease in absenteeism and staff turnover, and significant increases in productivity and morale. Characteristics of successful health promotion programmes include systematic organisation; availability to all staff; support from management; tailoring programmes to the specific needs of the organisation; good levels of resources; and continuation of programmes for a long time, rather than one-off initiatives. One of the major issues that needs to be faced and tackled is the balance between individual and organisational action. Programmes which emphasise the need for individuals to change, rather than also addressing policies and practices in the workplace, are less likely to be effective (Webb *et al.*, 1988). The lifestyle approach should be seen only as part of a more comprehensive approach to health promotion in the workplace.

References

Alexy, B. B. (1991). Factors associated with participation or non participation in a workplace wellness centre *Research in Nursing and Health*. *14*(1), 33–40.

Allinson, T., Cooper, C. L. & Reynolds, P. (1989). Stress counselling in the workplace: the Post Office experience. *The Psychologist* (September), *2*, 384–388.

Anon (1990). Polaroid: A health promotion programme for the workplace and the community. *Occupational Health Review*, *24*, 2–4.

Arroba, T. & James, K. (1990). Reducing the costs of stress: an organisational model. *Personnel Review*, *19*(1), 21–27.

Ashton, D. (1989). *The Corporate Health Care Revolution*. London: IPM/Kogan Page.

Batlle, E., Boixet, M., Agudo, A., Almirall, J. & Salvador, T. (1991). Tobacco prevention in hospitals: long-term follow-up of a smoking control programme. *British Journal of Addiction*, *86*, 709–717.

Batten, L. (1988). The NHS as agent of change: creating a smoke-free environment in hospitals. *Health Trends*, 20, 70–75.

Batten, L. (1990). *Managing Change: Smoking Policies in the NHS*. London: Health Education Authority.

Bovell, V. (1992). The economic benefits of health promotion in the workplace. In *Action on Health at Work Seminar*, 18 February 1992. London: Health Education Authority.

Bunce, D. & West, M. (1993). *Stress Management and Innovation Interventions at Work*. MRC/ESRC Social and Applied Psychology Unit, Memo Number 1359, University of Sheffield.

Clarkson, J., Blower, E., Hunter, C., Scale, I. & Nutbeam, D. (1991). *Overview of Innovative Workplace Action for Health in the UK*. European Foundation for the Improvement of Living and Working Conditions, working paper no: WP/91/03/EN.

Cooper, C. L. & Payne, R. (1988). *Causes, Coping and Consequences of Stress at Work*. New York & London: John Wiley.

Cooper, C. L. & Sadri, G. (1991). The impact of stress counselling at work. In P. L. Perewe (ed.), Handbook on Job Stress (special issue). *Journal of Social Behaviour and Personality*, *6*(7), 411–423.

Creed, F. (1993). Mental health problems at work. *British Medical Journal* (24 April), *306*, 1082–1083.

Defrank, R. S. & Cooper, C. L. (1987). Worksite stress management interventions: their effectiveness and conceptualisation. *Journal of Managerial Psychology*, 2, 4–10.

Department of Health (1992). *Creating Effective Smoking Policies in the NHS.* London : Health Education Authority.

Department of Health and Social Security (1988). *Fourth Report of the Independent Scientific Committee on Smoking and Health.* Chairman: Sir Peter Froggatt. London: HMSO.

Eriksen, M. P. (1988). Cancer prevention in workplace health promotion. *American Association of Occupational Health Nursing Journal*, *36*(6), 266–270.

Hallett, R. (1986). Smoking intervention in the workplace: review and recommendations. *Preventive Medicine*, 15 (3), 213–231.

Harvey, S. (1988). *Just an Occupational Hazard? Policies for Health at Work.* London: King's Fund Institute.

Health Education Authority (1988). *Stress in the Public Sector. Nurses, Police, Social Workers and Teachers.* London: Health Education Authority.

Health Education Authority (1990). *Action Plan on Stress.* London: HEA.

Health Education Authority (1991a). *Report on Qualitative Research to Inform Development of Cancer Education Programmes in the Workplace.* London: HEA.

Health Education Authority (1992a). *Action on Health at Work.* Report of a seminar, 18 February 1992. London: HEA.

Health Education Authority (1992b). *Health at Work in the NHS. Action Pack.* London : HEA.

Health Education Authority (1992c). *Health at Work in the NHS. Report on National Consultative Workshops.* London: HEA.

Health Education Authority (1993). *Health Promotion in the Workplace. A Summary.* London: HEA.

Hurst, T. (1992). *Towards a Smoke-Free Health Service. The 2nd Report.* Tom Hurst.

Industrial Relations Service (1989a). Health promotion at work. Parts 1 and 2. *Industrial Relations Service Employment Trends* (April & July), *438* and *443*.

Industrial Relations Service (1989b). Workplace health promotion at Polaroid. *Industrial Relations Service Employment Trends*, *454*, 11–14.

Industrial Relations Service (1992a). Smoking at work. Part 1. Why and how employers introduce smoking policies. *Industrial Relations Service Review and Report* (February), *506*, February, 4–10.

Industrial Relations Service (1992b). Smoking at work. Part 2. Policy content, growth and balance. *Industrial Relations Service Review and Report* (March) *507*, 5–13.

Jee, M. & Reason, L. (1988). *Action on Stress at Work.* London: Health Education Authority.

Jenkins, M., McEwan, J., Moreton, W. J., East, R., Seymour, L. & Goodin, M. (1987). *Smoking Policies at Work.* London : Health Education Authority.

Jenkins, R. & Coney, N. (1992). *Prevention of Mental Ill Health at Work. A Conference.* London: HMSO.

Klimes, I. (1989). *Promoting Well-Being at Work: Health Service Staff in Oxfordshire.* Oxford: Oxfordshire Department of Clinical Psychology.

Lovato, C. Y. & Green, L. W. (1990). Maintaining employee participation in workplace health promotion programs. *Health Education Quarterly, 17*(1), 73–88.

Matheson, H. (1987). *Health Promotion in the Workplace*. Scottish Health Education Group.

Murphy, L. R. (1988). Workplace intervention for stress reduction and prevention. In C. Cooper & R. Payne (eds), *Causes, Coping and Consequences of Stress at Work*. London & New York: J Wiley.

National Association for Staff Support (1992). *The costs of stress and the costs and benefits of stress management*. London: NASS.

Owen, G. M. (1993). *Taking the Strain. Stress, Coping Mechanisms and Support Systems for Professional Carers*. Literature Review, 4th edn. London: NASS.

Payne, R. & Firth-Cozens, J. (1987). *Stress in Health Professionals*. Chichester: John Wiley.

Pencack, M. (1991). Workplace health promotion programs. An overview. *Nursing Clinics of North America, 26*(1), 233–240.

Philo, J., Russell, J. & Pettersson, G. (1992). *Health at Work: A Needs Assessment in South West Thames Regional Health Authority*. London: South West Thames Regional Health Authority.

Rost, K. (1990). Predictors of employee involvement in a worksite health promotion program. *Health Education Quarterly, 17*(4), 395–407.

Sanders, D (1993). *Workplace Health Promotion. A Review of the Literature*. Oxford: Directorate of Health Policy and Public Health, Oxford Regional Health Authority.

Schilling, R. S. F. (1989). Health protection and promotion at work. *British Journal of Industrial Medicine, 46*(10), 683–688.

Trent Regional Health Authority (1993). *Health at Work in the NHS. A Directory of Current Practice in Trent*. Trent RHA.

Warner, K. E., Wickizer, T. M., Wolfe, R. A., Schildroth, J. E. & Samuelson, M. H. (1988). Economic implication of workplace health promotion programs: a review of the literature. *Journal of Occupational Medicine, 30* (2), 106–112.

Watson, N. (1992). *Provision of Employee Health and Welfare Programmes in a Range of Private and Public Sector Organisations in the UK*. Sunderland: University of Sunderland.

Webb, T., Schilling, R., Jacobson, B. & Babb, P. (1988). *Health at Work? A Report on Health Promotion at the Workplace*. Research Report No. 22. London: Health Education Authority.

19 *Alliances for health at work: a case study*

Miriam Glover

As outlined in the previous chapter, the workplace setting offers many opportunities to promote health and prevent disease. This chapter explores the role of healthy alliances in promoting health at work. The underlying premise presented is that alliances between relevant professionals are crucial to effect change for health in the workplace setting. Some of the opportunities for, and constraints on, partnership and cooperation between organisations aiming to promote health at work will be discussed. A major focus will be the way in which alliance partners can be involved in determining and implementing health policy at local level in the context of the workplace setting. Consequently, this chapter does not examine detailed studies of individual workplaces, references for these may be found in existing reviews of literature on the effectiveness of workplace health promotion (see, for example, Bovell, 1992 and Sanders, 1993).

Case Study of a Work Place Health Promotion Alliance

The Good Health Somerset workplace health promotion project was originally set up with a brief relating to lifestyle risk factors for coronary heart disease. The project has grown in response to local demand and *The Health of the Nation* (Department of Health, 1992). It currently offers an extensive portfolio of services encompassing health education, prevention and health protection measures. The project facilitator acts as a broker, forming links between local workplaces and organisations providing workplace health services. The project aims to support positive change for health at three levels within the workplace. The first of these is individual lifestyle change, the second is change in the working environment and the third is organisational change.

Since the workplace project was established, it has worked with more than half of the 169 largest employers in the county, those with more than 100 employees. Just over 25 per cent of the total county workforce of 167 000 are employed by 20 employers and 17 of these organisations have had substantial involvement with the project. The number of employees covered by the workplace programme is in excess of 40 000. (Figures taken from 1991 Census of Employment data supplied by the Environment Department, Somerset County Council and audit of Good Health Somerset project data.)

Planning and target setting

At the beginning of the project, identifying potential alliance partners was achieved largely through a process of trial and error. However, a number of motivated individuals were found who helped to plan the project and agreed to give it support. These included individuals from the County Council, District Councils and a trade union representative nominated by the South West TUC.

Developing commitment

With a small number of individual alliance partners it was straightforward to find common ground, link agendas and agree a plan. Building on the individuals' enthusiasm without gaining a formal commitment from the organisation they represented created a problem. Consequently, when there were changes of personnel, commitment to the project was lost and support had to be renegotiated with the individual's successor.

Concurrently, a number of factors contributed to a rise in profile of health at work at national level. These include the increase in workplace health and safety legislation from the European Union and, most recently, change in employers' contributions to statutory sick pay. At the local level, it has been interesting to note how information about the workplace project has spread by word of mouth through local employers' networks.

With time, the role of alliance partners in developing policy for promoting health at work has grown, not least from the impetus provided by *The Health of the Nation* to establish more formal alliances. The task of implementing local target setting in Somerset was given to the Health Promotion Strategic Planning Team working on behalf of the Joint Consultative Committee (JCC). Membership of this group is drawn from the Health Authority, Family Health Service Authority, Community Health Council, County Council and District Councils. Setting local targets presented a prime opportunity to consult local employers about setting some specific process targets for workplaces. For example, 60 per cent of employers with more than

100 employees will have a written smoking policy by 1995 and 75 per cent by 2000 (Somerset Health Promotion Strategic Planning Team, 1992).

The consultation process built on the already well-established workplace programme. The process is a good example of the moderate level of community participation in planning adapted from Brager and Sprecht (1973) outlined in Ewles and Simnett (1992, p. 193). In addition to private-sector workplaces, the target-setting process allowed the workplace programme to gain a greater and more formal commitment from public-sector employers, particularly the NHS and local authorities in Somerset. Specific public-sector process targets were agreed that recognised the health promotion role of the public sector with both staff and clients. These have been structured into strategies for implementation agreed at council meetings and meetings of the Health Authority board.

Monitoring public and private sector health promotion initiatives

Public and private workplace process targets are being monitored by a series of surveys. These provide information on progress for the Health Authority. They also provide an opportunity for the early dialogue over target setting to continue. For example, a 70 per cent response rate was achieved in the most recent postal questionnaire sent to workplaces with more than 100 employees. Many respondents requested a copy of the survey results, giving the Health Authority an excellent opportunity to maintain communication with the organisations involved. Analysis of the survey indicates that we have already exceeded the initial process targets set for the introduction of workplace smoking and alcohol policies in the private sector.

Mismatch between individual and organisational agendas

The JCC and its associated strategic planning team structure in Somerset has enabled many alliances supporting health promotion to be formalised. The structure has also given officers in the NHS and local authorities in the county an avenue to voice opinion and contribute to local policy development.

The major difficulty experienced, that has still to be addressed, is the dichotomy often found between the individual's interpretation of their organisation's values and policies and the party-line from the organisation itself. This problem is in part due to poor communication within organisations, but not solely. It arises from the way in which individuals function in organisations, the individual versus organisational agenda and power in organisations. Being aware of this issue is one way of coping with it. Another is to seek out the relevant representative of an organisation for the task in question. For example, if an alliance is being created to set policy an individual is required with enough power in their organisation to make a commitment to the policy that will be followed through.

The commissioning and enabling role

The second dimension for alliances is through the use of the commissioning role of health authorities and the enabling role of local authorities in support of their jointly agreed strategy to promote health at work. Since 1991 Somerset Health Authority's service specifications have included requirements for all contract holders to promote the health of staff and clients. This practice is widely used in other authorities. Killoran (1992, p. 4) claims that service specifications for health promotion and disease prevention have a tendency to include a requirement on all provider units to provide certain standards in relation to the quality of patient care; for example, a smoke-free environment and a requirement to promote the health of NHS employees. In Somerset, the Health Authority also have a specification for the Good Health Somerset workplace project. This includes support for the NHS in Somerset in developing health at work initiatives for staff. A further specification for community health services is to purchase a set amount of staff time each year for training in workplace health promotion and to carry that work out. This implies, in effect, that these NHS staff can use some of their time to promote health in their own workplace.

The contract dimension of alliance work is not confined to the NHS. Changes in local authorities and the introduction of their enabling role has led to a similar use of service specifications. For example, the specification for a leisure facility may include the requirement that staff and clients are covered by a smoking policy. The commissioning/enabling route to support workplace health promotion does have limitations. A specification cannot dictate how a provider organisation should manage its staff or detail what an organisational culture should be. These are two important factors in determining health at work. However this route is an additional way of formalising a commitment to promoting health at work and can give alliance partners an opportunity to be prescriptive about issues such as working environments. The inclusion of even the most basic requirements in a specification can open the door to more detailed discussions of health at work, and certainly helps to raise the profile of workplace health promotion. Very often, requirements can be extended to cover users of a service as well as the staff providing it, a theme that will be returned to later.

Providing workplace services

The workplace facilitator acts as a broker putting workplaces in contact with the relevant public, private or voluntary organisation which is best placed to support them. For example, when introducing an alcohol policy, a workplace may wish to access counselling services for employees which can be provided by a local voluntary agency. While marketing workplace health promotion services in a company, a query about occupational health may arise. This would be dealt with by putting the company in touch with the local NHS occupational health service.

An effective working partnership between so many professional groups is not easy to create. In order to maintain harmony, clear boundaries are negotiated. This involves identifying what service an individual or organisation is best qualified to provide and then encouraging people to stick within their remit. The process is helped by having the workplace facilitator acting as a central coordinator. The facilitator markets services to the workplace, works with the company to identify health needs and negotiates a service from the relevant agency on behalf of the workplace.

Charging workplaces for services is an issue that could potentially be a problem within the provider alliance. The majority of workplaces have no budget for health promotion (Health Education Authority, 1992a), and the very few that have money to spend do not have much. Often the services from other public and voluntary bodies are available to workplaces free of charge or at low cost. A requirement to raise income from workplace health promotion would put strain on alliance relationships and increase competition between alliance members.

The partnership of providers is also helped by having *The Health of the Nation* local targets and strategies agreed between the major public sector professionals, as discussed earlier. This gives broad terms of reference for individual or professional responsibilities.

Workplaces themselves contribute to the provider alliance. For example, a number of local companies have run promotional events for the project by inviting other workplaces in their area for a lunch and briefing session. Other employers have hosted and contributed to training days on issues such as stress at work. Some workplaces have worked with us to pilot new services. For example, a sexual-health exhibition for a local company was run jointly between Good Health Somerset, the local family planning service and two occupational health nurses from the company.

The workplace as a health promoter in its own right

This final dimension to working in partnership could be seen as the ultimate alliance. The ideal is for a workplace to consider and act upon staff health issues and then turn their attention to promoting health outside the organisation, through the products and/or services they offer.

The Health Education Authority's (HEA) 'Look After Your Heart' workplace programme involves employers signing up to a minimum of three points on a workplace charter. Point 10 of the charter states that the workplace will 'Explore with the HEA opportunities to work on the development and promotion of health, healthy products and services' (HEA, 1992b, p. 6).

Public sector workplaces are more likely to be in a position to consider their wider health promotion role than the private sector. The involvement of both the NHS and local authorities in implementing *The Health of the Nation* at local level, as described earlier, has allowed them to develop the notion of health promotion beyond working with staff. Examples include the introduction of policies on issues such as smoking that not only protect staff from environmental tobacco smoke but also create smoke-free public places.

Opportunities for this type of work with private-sector companies are more limited. When companies are in business to make a profit they are reluctant to give serious consideration to changing their products or services unless they are going to realise a substantial return. One representative of a brewing company gave an excellent account of his company's efforts to promote staff health at the 1993 Association of Public Health conference. The rationale he put forward was that it made sound business sense to promote staff health, reflected in the low absenteeism in the company and their low accident rates. However, when asked by a member of the audience 'would the company ever be prepared to discuss the health impact of their products?', the answer was a firm 'no'.

The ideal of encouraging workplaces to become health promoters in their own right is laudable. The corporatist lobby can be a powerful one in helping to shape policy. However, when influencing health policy this lobby can often be negative rather than positive. Ham (1992) cites the example of the way in which the National Advisory Committee on Nutrition Education (NACNE) guidelines on health and nutrition were opposed by the food industry. The example of the negative impact of the tobacco industry on health policy is cited in Downie *et al.* (1990) and is well documented in other sources.

Nonetheless, there are developments in management in some companies that give grounds for hope. The issue of social responsibility is gaining a higher profile in some workplaces. MacIntosh (1993) lists a number of components of the social responsibility agenda which include concern for the environment, equal opportunities and health and safety amongst many others. He argues that there is a shift in the way employers are dealing with these issues. Some organisations are developing a notion of social responsibility that is threading through their business operations. This early work on corporate social responsibility is encouraging but more study of this area is required.

This chapter has attempted to show how one local workplace health promotion project has put alliance-working into practice at both the strategic and operational level. The discussion has highlighted the need for an agreed strategic approach in order to provide a foundation for joint work.

Employers are an important alliance partner. Public sector workplaces inevitably are more closely involved in local policy processes than those in the private sector. Establishing mechanisms for dialogue with the workplace health professionals is key. The implementation of *The Health of the Nation* at local level provides one route into this.

Ultimately, the workplace is just one setting of many where health promotion activities can be targeted. While support for staff health activities appears to be growing, the workplace, particularly in the private sector, offers only limited opportunities for promoting health in the wider community. Indeed, the interests of companies may well be invested in opposing policy measures at national level that would promote health. A small body of evidence from the study of the social responsibility agenda in companies indicates the possibility for change, but this early work is far from conclusive.

There is real potential for optimising the promotion of health at work, utilising a healthy alliance approach. These approaches must be tempered, however, by a realistic appreciation of what this potential is, and how it might best be optimised.

References

Bovell, V. (1992). *The Economic Benefits of Health Promotion in the Workplace.* London: Health Education Authority.

Downie, R., Fyfe, C. & Tannahill, A. (1990). *Health Promotion: Models and Values.* Oxford: Oxford University Press.

Ewles, L. & Simnett, I. (1992). *Promoting Health: A Practical Guide*, 2nd edn. London: Scutari.

Ham, C. (1992). *Health Policy in Britain*, 3rd edn. London: Macmillan.

Health Education Authority (1992a). *Health At Work Survey*. London: HEA.

Health Education Authority (1992b). *Working for a Healthier Future*, 2nd edn. London: Health Education Authority.

Department of Health (1992). *The Health of the Nation*. London: HMSO.

Killoran, A. (1992). *Putting Health Into Contracts*. London: Health Education Authority.

MacIntosh, M. (1993). *Good Business? Case Studies in Corporate Social Responsibility*. Bristol: School of Advanced Urban Studies.

Sanders, D. (1993). *Workplace Health Promotion: A Review of the Literature*. Oxford: Oxford Regional Health Authority.

20 Trade unions and health promotion

Marc Beishon and Sarah Veale

In recent years, trade unions have become important agents in helping to initiate and sustain workplace health promotion. During the 1980s and 1990s, many unions have developed their traditional health and safety functions to cover pressing workplace health issues such as work-related upper-limb disorders and stress, as well as cooperating with employers in broader campaigns such as cancer screening, healthier eating, and initiatives to cut the consumption of tobacco, alcohol and drugs (Health Education Authority, 1992).

It is important to recognise that one of the primary roles of trade unions has always been to ensure that employees are working in safe and healthy conditions (Trades Union Congress, 1992). But unions see this role as part of a democratic process of collective bargaining, not as a direct appeal to interfere with the rights and choices of an individual. Unions concentrate on socioeconomic factors that can be negotiated with employers, not lifestyle issues.

Acknowledging this distinction is crucial to gaining the cooperation of unions in workplace healthy alliances. However, with the long-standing concern for industrial health and safety issues, unions have begun to adopt the view that it is inconsistent to separate certain health issues from the more traditional shop-floor emphasis on safety. The Trades Union Congress (TUC) has always maintained that the two are inseparable (Trades Union Congress, 1992). For example, it would be inconsistent to provide healthy eating options in the staff canteen if workers were then expected to return to a shop floor with dangerously high noise levels.

Some so-called health promotion initiatives are viewed with great suspicion by unions (Trades Union Congress, 1992). There have been some thinly-veiled attempts to weed out less healthy employees for redundancy. But in a context of full consultation, and a consistent health and safety policy across an organisation, unions are not likely to be hostile to health promotion activities.

Background to trade unions

Today in Britain there are 69 trade unions affiliated to the TUC, representing more than 7.5 million members (Trades Union Congress, 1992). There are trade union members in every industry and service, including top managers, scientists, teachers, printers, skilled workers, labourers, radiographers, musicians and airline pilots.

Part-time workers are increasing as a proportion of trade unionists in employment, and the current union density, that is the number of workers in unions, is overall about 35 per cent of the total workforce (Department of Employment, 1994).

Unions are organised in different ways, depending on their size and the type of employee they represent. A large union, such as the General, Municipal and Boilermakers Union (GMB) has a national office with departments covering different services and trade groups, and a number of regional offices staffed by full-time officials. The GMB has more than 40 national health and safety officers. A small union such as the Communication Managers' Association has no regional offices (Trades Union Congress, 1994b).

Most unions also have a large number of lay officers, those not employed by the union but who undertake certain duties in the workplace, such as health and safety representatives. In total, there are about 2000 full-time union officers, the majority of whom work for the large unions. There are more than 90 000 lay safety representatives in Britain, and more than 70 per cent of working people have access to one of these volunteer officials (Trades Union Congress, 1992).

Since the Health and Safety at Work Act 1974, safety representatives have become an integral part of the management of health and safety at the workplace, with rights to investigate accidents, inspect the workplace and to be consulted by the employer about health and safety training programmes and the introduction of new production methods or machinery into the workplace. Inspectors from the Health and Safety Executive (HSE) also talk to union safety representatives when carrying out their inspections and may discuss their findings with them. The TUC trains more than 7000 safety representatives each year in setting up effective health and safety committees. A number of larger unions have a health and safety committee made up of national executive members.

With more than 700 people dying each year in workplace accidents (Trades Union Congress, 1992), 170 000 major injuries and an estimated 10 000 deaths as a result of work-related health damage, it is hardly surprising that safety and certain direct health hazards are a priority for unions. For example, the TUC recommends that safety committees check health records on absenteeism, referrals to the occupational health department, data on biological monitoring, hearing tests, the causes of death of past employees and the results of surveys seeking out specific health problems, such as lower-back pain, skin problems, respiratory complaints, work-related upper-limb disorders and symptoms of stress (Trades Union Congress, 1994a).

At national level, health and safety is one of the few remaining areas which is conducted on a tripartite basis, with Government, employers and union representatives working together to develop national health and safety policies and legislation. Trade unions in other countries have similar concerns about health and safety in the workplace, with varying degrees of statutory support (Trades Union Congress, 1994a).

Table 20.1 shows the representation of unions in various occupations; Table 20.2 shows that the vast majority of union membership is in organisations with at least 25 employees. Overall, about 40 per cent of the British workforce is employed by small businesses with mostly low pay, no union representation and little access to workplace health initiatives (Trades Union Congress, 1994b).

Table 20.1   *Union density by type of occupation (1991)*

Type of occupation	Union density(%)
Professional occupations	52
Associate professional and technical occupations	50
Plant and machine operatives	50
Craft and related occupations	46
Other occupations	36
Personal and protective service occupations	32
Clerical and secretarial occupations	31
Managers and administrators	25
Sales occupations	15
All persons	37

Source: Trades Union Congress, 1992 Report to Congress. Reproduced with the permission of the TUC.

Table 20.2   *Union density by size of workplace (1991)*

Number of workers in workplace	Number of workers covered	Density (%)
Fewer than 6 employees	2.5 million	11
6–24 employees	1.16 million	23
25 or more employees	14.34 million	47

Source: Trades Union Congress, 1992 Report to Congress. Reproduced with the permission of the TUC.

Health promotion

Health promotion began to interest some unions as a concept in its own right at the beginning of the 1990s, as the Government prepared to launch *The Health of the Nation* White Paper. It also became clear during the recent recession that the vast majority of absence from work was through sickness, not industrial action or other reasons (Department of Health, 1992). This prompted many employers to pay increasing attention to health issues, while some unions, particularly in the white-collar sector, have recognised that promoting healthier workplaces can add to the package of services and support on offer to members.

Some issues, such as smoking and alcohol misuse, are both safety and lifestyle issues and are not new as workplace concerns. The Manufacturing, Science and Finance Union (MSF), for example, has had a model smoking agreement in place for use by negotiators for some time (Manufacturing, Science and Finance Union, undtated). The Civil and Public Services Association (CPSA) has also negotiated many smoking agreements, often using ballots of members (Civil and Public Service Association, 1994). The CPSA points out that it gets involved in negotiating new policies, but it is the employers responsibility to operate them.

There are some relatively new areas of concern which have a health promotion aspect as well as a more traditional context. One is stress or mental health in the workplace, which includes issues such as bullying and violence to staff. Another is work-related upper-limb disorder, formerly known as repetitive strain injury (RSI). Although not a new issue, it has only recently been addressed by most unions; the National Union of Journalists and a few others have been researching RSI since the early 1980s. The TUC has run a successful campaign which not only aims to claim compensation for such injuries, but also aims to make changes in the workplace and the job so that injuries no longer occur (Trades Union Congress, 1994a).

In 1992, the Health Education Authority carried out a survey covering more than 1000 organisations in the public and private sectors (Health Education Authority, 1993). The aim was to find out whether health promotion issues were on the agenda and, if so, how much importance was attached to them.

Significant factors indicating the likely presence of workplace health promotions such as smoking and alcohol policies included both a larger organisation size and the presence of a recognised trade union. For example, about two-fifths (41 per cent) of workplaces with a union were found to have a smoking-related activity, compared with 28 per cent of cases with no union (Health Education Authority, 1993).

Approaches to health promotion

There are plenty of large-scale initiatives by employers, particularly in the private sector, where consultation with unions has eased the introduction of health promotion initiatives. However, there are few well-documented examples, and it is unusual to find action initiated by unions purely on the grounds of health promotion. Most of the examples where more information is available are in the public sector, particularly in the transport area.

British Rail (BR) is a case in point. In some respects, its introduction of a tough policy on drugs and alcohol, prompted by the Transport and Works Act 1992, can be seen as having a health promotion aspect (Beishon, 1994). BR's policy is driven by safety. It requires that no staff report to work while unfit through the use of drugs or alcohol, and forbids their consumption while at work. Staff face dismissal and possible prosecution if tested positive for alcohol and drugs.

While welcoming BR's initiative, railway unions such as the Transport Salaried Staffs Association (TSSA) have been concerned about the legalistic way in which such regimes have been introduced and enforced. The view is that a punitive, rather than educational, approach misses opportunities to promote healthier options in a wider sense, and is less likely to gain the full cooperation of staff.

For example, an alcohol and drugs policy that includes a comprehensive counselling, amnesty and education programme from the outset is likely to be more successful. Unions want to have joint ownership of the introduction of these measures, and in BRs case, unions have worked hard to increase the occupational facilities made available by the company for services such as welfare counselling. In circulars to members, the TSSA urges members to come forward if they have a problem, but promises to defend anyone treated unfairly by the new procedures.

One company that has won praise from all quarters for its consultation procedures is Parcelforce, the distribution company within the Post Office, which has health promotion policies on smoking, alcohol, HIV/AIDS and general safety. It also encourages healthy eating and provides various health screening services. The company has noted the link between good health and productivity, and the cost of sickness. In setting up its smoking policy, the support was first gained from the board, then consultations were made with the various unions, addressing their concerns about the timescale for introducing the policy, support to be offered and enforcement.

Other initiatives have been more directly related to health promotion, such as a stress programme for London bus drivers and a heart disease prevention exercise at London Underground (Coronary Prevention Group, 1993). These projects succeeded only with the coop-eration of unions. Important agents in implementations are bodies such as the Health Education Authority, with its Look After Your-self/Look After Your Heart tutor-led programme, the Coronary Pre-vention Group, Alcohol Concern and Action on Smoking and Health ASH. The train driver's union, ASLEF, has carried out work with the Coronary Prevention Group on alcohol and smoking in the work-place.

Where a union does take direct action it is usually a specific work-place campaign, such as persuading management to provide healthier food in hospital canteens for longer hours, rather than force staff to rely on vending machines.

Stress is on the agenda of many unions. There is a feeling that it is the issue of the 1990s, like RSI in the 1980s. The union approach to stress is to concentrate on those factors that are in the control of employers, such as child-care facilities for hard-pressed parents, and improvements to the environment. Although stress has often been linked with highly-paid executives, they tend to have more control over their working conditions. Only lately has it been more fully appreciated that workers such as nurses, who have a far more rigid regime, suffer very high stress levels.

This approach is consistent with the traditional union approach to safety issues, and is also driven by demands of members at a particu-lar time. White-collar unions are also involved in long-running cam-paigns on the use of visual-display units.

The Health of the Nation

The TUC welcomed the inclusion of the workplace in *The Health of the Nation* White Paper as an important forum for health promotion, and is committed to working in the Governments Workplace Steering Group at the Department of Health. However, it criticised the paper for failing to make links between socioeconomic factors and ill-health, and also found inconsistencies in not banning cigarette advertising, in the lack of attention paid to food and alcohol labelling, and cuts in services such as school meals and family-planning services.

And of course accident prevention, long a union priority, is now directly relevant to health promotion as it is a key area in *The Health of the Nation*. The union standpoint is that about 90 per cent of all workplace accidents are preventable, and 70 per cent are directly attri-butable to the failure of an employers control systems. Given that responsibility for preventing most accidents in the workplace lies with the employer, unions have understandably been unhappy about the focus on the individual in *The Health of the Nation*. More attention, they feel, should be paid to the responsibility of employers under existing statutory duties. Also, as the NHS is the main agent for delivering the objectives of the White Paper, the TUC considers that under current funding constraints there is little that health authorities can do to find the additional resources needed to meet these objectives.

The TUC has argued that to be effective, health promotion initiatives in the workplace should follow proper consultation with the workforce. To be successful, the same treatment should be applied throughout the workplace. Executive gyms or selective smoking bans give the wrong message about health promotion. Programmes for women, such as cervical cancer screening are excellent, but programmes for men, for example on prostate screening, should also be included.

Anything that looks like coercion must be avoided, and programmes must not be negative in tone. For example, on diet the emphasis should be on how pleasant healthy foods are, not on the danger of fatty foods. Employers should not exaggerate or try too much at once. Nor should unions and employers confuse statutory requirements with voluntary measures.

Ideally, a joint committee of management and unions, either an existing health and safety committee, or a new health promotion committee, should adopt a strategic and systematic approach with achievable objectives and a proper review process.

Unions in industries such as the railways are facing the prospect of shrinking resources provided by employers, due to privatisation, and are concerned about the general erosion of peoples health. They are beginning to form a holistic picture of health and well-being as the pressure increases to work longer hours, under more stressful conditions, and often for a shrinking pay packet. Britons now work some of the longest hours in Europe (Department of Employment, 1994).

As ever, unions see their role as persuading employers to create better environments for workers, and health is likely to increase further in importance at the negotiating table in the latter half of the 1990s.

References

Beishon, M. (1994). Healthy negotiation: the union stance. *Healthlines*. February, no. 9.

Coronary Prevention Group (1993). *Annual Report*. London: CPG.

Civil and Public Services Association (1993). *Model Smoking Agreement*. London: CPSA.

Department of Employment (1994). *Labour Force Survey*. London: HMSO.

Department of Health (1992). *The Health of the Nation*. London: HMSO.

Health Education Authority (1992). *Health Promotion in the Workplace: The Trades Union Movement*. London: HEA.

Health Education Authority (1993). *Health Promotion in the Workplace: A Summary*. London: HEA.

Manufacturing, Science and Finance Union (undated). *Smoking at Work: Negotiating a Policy*. MSF Health and Safety Information, *140*, 25.

Trades Union Congress (1992). *Response to The Health of the Nation*. London: TUC.

Trades Union Congress (1994a). *Better Safety Standards at Work*. London: TUC.

Trades Union Congress (1994b). *Report to 1994 Congress*. London: TUC.

21 The role of occupational health services in promoting health

Jennifer Lisle

The working population is a key group within society, comprising 24 million people in the UK and some 350 million in the European region. The working population is therefore a very major target group for health promotion.

Workplace health promotion has the potential to reach large numbers of people but needs to be considered within the changing context of work. Throughout the 1980s and continuing through the 1990s, the rapid pace of change has continued to produce a great deal of turbulence and uncertainty in the workplace. Work environments have altered enormously as a result of the new technologies which have radically changed work practices for people in all types of organisations. Patterns of work and working hours have changed, the pace of work has also accelerated. Competition has increased as markets have become global and there continues to be a relentless drive for greater efficiency and increased productivity (Lisle, 1991).

In the UK and in many other European countries, there has been a large increase in the number of people working in the service industries with a corresponding decline in those working in manufacturing industry. In Britain, over two-thirds of those employed are now working in service industries. There has been a marked trend away from full-time male employment with a significant increase in the number of part-time workers, particularly women, and in service industry shift work (Office of Population Censuses and Surveys, 1992). It is hardly surprising that job insecurity is now commonplace, and that uncertainty about the future is a fact for many industries and their workforces. Even the previously secure industries such as banking and insurance have been shaken by the rapidity of change. Companies face the ever-present possibility of mergers and takeovers and are no longer able to give guarantees of lifelong careers to their employees.

A pattern of redundancy and unemployment, frequent job change and an increasing need for mobility is emerging as the twentieth century draws to an end. Changes of this magnitude affecting the values, concepts, beliefs and norms of society have been described by

Kuhn (1970) as paradigm shifts, fundamental changes in the basic patterns.

The current situation requires a new health paradigm to fulfil the changing views and needs of society. There is growing awareness and an urgent need to place more emphasis on the environment and ecological issues. Organisations are beginning to recognise their responsibility to develop new strategies in order to address these global environmental problems. They also have an opportunity to create a different kind of workplace which could play an important part in the development of a new approach to health.

The World Health Organisation's (WHO) Regional Director for Europe (Asvall, 1991, p. 53) has pointed out that as the stability of organisations is threatened by rapidly changing markets, their ability to survive requires much more than approaches used in the past:

> Today we require a courageous change in attitudes, a more open communication between workers and management and a new willingness to enter into a real dialogue and to share more seriously the responsibility for finding solutions that are acceptable both to workers and to management.

The infrastructure of the workplace is continually changing with the current tendency to decentralisation and fragmentation of the larger organisations. There are problems of access to the very large numbers of small workplaces where labour turnover is high. Such factors present an enormous challenge for occupational health provision; how to design services which will meet the health needs of so many different types of workforce.

Occupational health provision

Many European countries have given high priority to occupational health services in their general health policies. However, occupational health services in Europe vary considerably and there are major differences between countries. For example, in Finland, Norway, France and Germany, occupational health services are a statutory part of their health-care systems; but in other countries, for example Britain, the responsibility rests with individual employers. In the UK there is no statutory regulation requiring any occupational health service other than first aid to be provided in-house for the workforce. It tends to be the larger organisations which provide occupational health services for their employees, but only about half of the UK workforce has access to a health professional at work (Bunt 1993).

The National Health Service (NHS) is the largest employer in

Europe, and its role as a leader in workplace health promotion should be exemplary. NHS workplace health policies affect patient care. Therefore, policies must ensure safe work practices, including the organisation of work, which will benefit the health of employees and hence their ability to care effectively for patients. The NHS Management Executive commissioned the Health Education Authority to develop Health at Work in the NHS (1992). This long-term initiative aims to ensure that the NHS in England provides healthy workplaces and so contributes to the health and well-being of its employees and the public they serve. It is complementary to other initiatives such as Health Promoting Hospitals (1994), Opportunity 2000, Investors in People and Look After Your Heart (LAYH), which seek to enhance the health and well-being of NHS employees.

Occupational health policies: a comprehensive approach

Many organisations have only minimal policies on Health and Safety with no specific occupational health policy; existing guidelines on occupational health services are often outdated. Occupational health policies need to be more comprehensive to include not only health protection but also health promotion and psychosocial issues. So far, very little has been done to create policies to protect or promote the psychological health of the workforce. A survey of occupational health services in Europe by the World Health Organisation (1990) showed that psychological provision in the workplace is still very limited, although a number of countries mentioned psychological hazards as targets for activity.

A comprehensive approach therefore aims at not only preventing injuries and illness but at actively promoting health. Health policies need to encompass this proactive dimension. Within individual organisations the links between the physical and mental health of the workforce must be understood by management. In order to be healthy an organisation needs to develop health policies which address both physical and psychological problems encountered in the work environment. The aim should be to create a work environment supportive of positive health practices based on a belief that a healthy organisation requires healthy employees and that merely urging employees to take more responsibility for their health and providing the opportunity for them to do so will not be effective without a supportive corporate culture.

The workplace should be a focus for the development and implementation of new health policies. The health of the working population is of vital importance to the economy as well as to the prosperity of local populations. The contemporary workplace and its workforce has become a crucial public health concern. Ensuring that new health policies in the workplace include both health protection and health promotion offers an opportunity to promote the health of a key sector of the population (Faculty of Public Health Medicine, 1995).

Improving health in the workplace

The workplace is an important setting for preventive activities and since people spend about one-third of their waking hours at work, the workplace has considerable potential for health promotion. It has a key role to play in achieving Health for All targets (World Health Organisation, 1993) and the four main objectives:

- Greater equity in health;
- The promotion and facilitation of healthy lifestyles;
- A reduction in the burden of preventable ill health;
- A re-orientation of health care systems.

It is increasingly difficult to distinguish between illness caused by work and illness due to other causes. There are no clear boundaries and many health problems develop over a long time scale and have multiple causes, for example cardiovascular disease. This broader view of occupational health allows for factors related to lifestyle to be tackled; for example, alcohol and drug abuse (Schilling, 1989). The overall aim is to promote the general health of workers, their physical, mental and social well-being, and to optimise working conditions so that work is better adapted to the workers, to both their physiological and psychological needs.

The overall aims of an occupational health policy should be:

- To provide a safe and healthy workplace;
- To promote optimal physical and mental/emotional health of all employees;
- To strengthen the relationship between health and productivity so that employees can contribute effectively to the organisation's goals and also enhance their own personal well-being.

In order to provide a safe and healthy workplace, *health protection* policies must cover the assessment of *health risk* both physical and psychological which could cause, aggravate or contribute to ill-health and which may lead to other problems; for example, sickness absence. *Assessment of fitness for work* requires consideration of the medical aspects of selection, job change, rehabilitation and ill-health retirement, while policies on occupational disease prevention must aim to identify at-risk groups, particularly those exposed to particular hazards, either physical or psychological (Edwards *et al.*, 1988).

Policies on *health promotion* should be developed alongside those on *health protection*. A proactive organisation will formulate specific policies on *alcohol and drug abuse, smoking, and prevention of stress* in relation to the management of change as well as policies aimed at heart disease prevention and *counselling* for employees with problems.

Policies need to be dynamic and project something positive; for example, that support for employees is vital whilst organisations are restructuring. Such policies will have a direct bearing on productivity and employee morale. Job satisfaction and efficiency are inseparable.

An adequate standard of health and safety provision is a prerequisite for workplace health promotion. Nothing will be gained by a superficial approach. Organisations need to make a genuine commitment to health, recognising that in looking beyond immediate short-term gains, they are building a sound foundation for the future.

Promoting mental health at work

In the UK, the Health and Safety Executive (1988), pointed out the value of instituting an occupational health policy which includes consideration of all aspects of mental health. There is increasing evidence that an unsatisfactory work environment may lead to psychological disorder. Karasek and Theorell (1990) have shown that it is not the demands of work itself but the organisational structure of work that plays the most consistent role in the development of stress related illness. Jobs that give workers little opportunity to make decisions or to decide which skills to use are wasteful of their actual capabilities. Adverse psychosocial factors are also risk factors for cardiovascular illness, providing an explanation for the higher mortality from coronary heart disease of workers in the lower social classes who are more likely to experience psychosocial stress at work. Policies should therefore be developed to address psychological job design and its health and productivity consequences.

Cox *et al.* (1990) suggest that organisational health is about more than the sum of the health of individual employees. Simply attempting to represent the health of an organisation in terms of employee health profiles (for example, blood pressure or cholesterol), is thus inadequate. The central idea is that the organisation offers a number of different environments to employees, the qualities of which are powerful predictors of important organisational issues such as staff turnover and absence, for example. It can be seen, therefore, that policies on health need to be considered alongside policies on employment, the work environment and as an integral part of company policy.

Occupational health services

An Occupational Health Service (OHS) is responsible for providing advice concerning the health of people at work. The cost is borne by the employer. In order to be effective throughout the organisation and in order to operate in a proactive way, occupational health services must have the commitment of the senior management and the board of a company. There should be corporate leadership on health to set the standards for health and communicate these to all levels of the organisation. The professional in charge of the OHS must also have access to the most senior level of management in the company, if required, and the occupational health team must be able to operate impartially at all levels of the organisation.

The OHS may include medical, nursing and occupational hygiene services plus contributions when required from other disciplines; for example, ergonomists and psychologists. The range of activities is broad, but the emphasis is on prevention rather than cure.

Relationship with employees

Employees must be able to view the OHS as a resource which they can use to resolve problems and difficulties, to seek advice and guidance so as to minimise the effect on their work performance without detriment to their jobs and career prospects. Unless the OHS is seen by employees to be impartial and confidential it will not have any credibility with them, thus negating its usefulness as a resource. This is particularly important with regard to mental health problems (Lisle, 1991).

An OHS should, however, collaborate to help management recognise situations which are potentially hazardous or stressful and to identify groups of employees at particular risk. The main functions of a well developed OHS (WHO, 1990) are as follows:

- Surveillance of the work environment;
- Initiatives and advice on the control of hazards at work;
- Surveillance of the health of employees;
- Follow-up of the health of vulnerable groups;
- Adaptation of work and the work environment to the worker;
- Organisation of first-aid and emergency response;
- Health education and health promotion;
- Collection of information on workers' health.

Although these activities have usually focused on the physical work environment, they apply equally to the psychological work environment and the mental health of employees. The occupational health activities listed meet the WHO and International Labour Organisation guidelines (International Labour Organisation, 1985). However, a World Health Organisation (1990) survey of Occupational Health Services showed that psychological and psychosocial aspects of occupational health in Europe had so far received little attention.

Types of occupational health service

Occupational health services are organised in various ways. At one end of the spectrum provision is limited to *First Aid* and *minor treatment services* provided at the workplace. Group services are independent services which provide for several workplaces in the same locality. They may serve a large number of small to medium size companies within an industrial estate, for example. Large organisations often have an *in-house OHS* which can provide a wide range of facilities and services. In Scandinavia there are *specialised* occupational health services for specific industries; for example, there is a nationwide service for the Swedish construction industry.

The planning of occupational health activities must start with identifying the needs of the organisation and the specific hazards in the workplace. Further requirements of an OHS are:

- To be an impartial, advisory, expert function;
- To work on a preventive basis;
- To be staffed by personnel trained for the purpose;
- To have competence and resources for vocational rehabilitation;
- To be integrated or coordinated with the firm's Health and Safety committees;
- To be user friendly.

Some ways in which an OHS can assist

Assessment and diagnosis of problems

This is especially important in connection with poor work performance and early identification of specific problems, for example alcohol dependency and stress, in individuals or groups of workers. There is a very large burden of minor mental health problems which largely go unnoticed since they do not result in referral to specialists, but which contribute significantly to poor work performance. The scope for health promotion in this area is enormous and has the potential to improve not only the health of an individual but also that of the organisation as a whole.

Assessment of fitness for work, rehabilitation

The assessment of long-term health problems are especially important. Liaison with an employee's own doctor is crucial in order that the occupational health adviser can provide essential guidance for management on fitness for work and rehabilitation.

Sickness absence

An OHS can analyse short and long-term absence and provide an assessment of individuals and groups which can lead to a reduction in absence, assisting managers to understand the underlying causes.

Monitoring 'at-risk' groups

It is important to monitor the health of people employed in certain hazardous jobs, and also groups such as shift workers. This facilitates early identification of health problems and action to safeguard employee well-being.

Counselling

There is much scope for both reactive and proactive counselling in the workplace, for example:

- For groups of employees experiencing organisational change or exposed to other stressful events;
- For individuals with stress, alcohol or work-related problems.

An OHS can assist employees by *initiating treatment* and *speeding up referral*.

Advice on the health effects of new work practices and new technologies

An OHS has a proactive role in giving employees simple practical advice on health issues arising from new work practices and technologies such as VDU/display screen work.

Health promotion

Workplace health promotion includes many of the traditional activities described above, but health promotion is a larger concept than is usually evident in traditional activities in that it does not differentiate between sources of threat to health which arise within the workplace and outside. Health promotion seeks to influence the health of individuals in a positive way regardless of the source of threat to health. Wynne (1990) and Wynne and Clarkin (1992) have described examples of good practice and innovation observed in different organisations and countries. An organisation's OHS has a central role to play in stimulating interest in health promotion and ensuring the continuity of health promotion programmes.

Other benefits of occupational health services

The presence of an occupational health team can bring about improvement in morale of a workforce, leading to greater efficiency and productivity, improved industrial relations and a positive attitude to health which contributes to a healthy workforce.

Links with other organisations

In order to be proactive in the health promotion field, the OHS needs to form links with many outside organisations and specialist resources. The OHS should not be a service in isolation but rather the centre of a network of services which can be made accessible to the organisation and bring to it a range of different skills.

The need for proactive occupational health services

The speed with which change is occurring in the workplace has produced a great deal of upheaval and uncertainty. In many organisations, particularly the rapidly growing service sector, mental health demands have escalated. Change is a challenge, a stimulus for new ideas but it is essential to understand the stressful effect it can have on employees. Often its effect is profound, affecting the health of the organisation as a whole and its ability to function effectively. Pressures in the workplace and in the marketplace are also having a considerable impact on occupational health services. Can they tackle these complex problems? For example, how relevant is the professional training to cope with mental health issues? New occupational health priorities are developing. If the needs of the changing workplace are to be met, occupational health services have to provide much more now than a decade ago.

Organisations need a new perception of occupational health professionals and the skills they can offer. In order to tackle problems there is a real need for the OHS to interact with the organisation it serves and to form appropriate alliances with organisations outside the workplace. The OHS should be a dynamic resource, playing a key role in organisational strategies to help create healthy, caring and successful organisations (Lisle, 1991).

Responsibility for improving the health of those at work is a joint responsibility of management, trade unions, government, health professionals and all employees. The old model of reacting to problems when they arise must be superseded by a much more proactive and dynamic approach. Preventive strategies for health, showing recognition of the connections between the physical and psychological health of the workforce and recognition of working conditions, including the psychosocial environment, are essential and should be part of the operating plan of every organisation.

Occupational health policy should not be drawn up in isolation but should form part of a coherent strategy for achieving *Health for All by the year 2000*. The workplace should be a focus for the development and implementation of new health policies which will be instrumental in the development of healthy organisations.

References

Asvall, J. E. (1991). Viewpoint '91. Health for all in Europe: challenge for health at work. *Occupational Medicine, 41*, 53–54.

Bunt, K. (1993). *Occupational Health Provision at Work*. Health and Safety Executive, Contract Research Report No. 57. London: HMSO.

Cox, T., Leather, P. & Cox, S. (1990). Stress, health and organisations. *Occupational Health Review, 23*, 13–18.

Edwards, F. C., McCallum, R. I. & Taylor, P. J. (eds) (1988). *Fitness for Work*. Oxford: Oxford University Press.

Faculty of Public Health Medicine (1995). Health Promotion in the Workplace, *Guidelines for Health Promotion Number 40*. London: Faculty of Public Health Medicine.

Health Education Authority (1993). *Health Promoting Hospitals: Principles and Practice*. London: HEA.

Health Education Authority and National Health Service Management Executive (1992). *Health at Work in the NHS - Action Pack*. London: HEA.

Health and Safety Executive (1988). *Mental Health at Work*. London: HMSO.

International Labour Organisation (1985). *Convention 161 and Recommendation 171 on Occupational Health Services*. London: ILO.

Karasek, R. & Theorell, T. (1990). *Healthy Work: Stress, Productivity and the Reconstruction of Working Life*. New York: Basic Books.

Kuhn, T. (1970). *The Structure of Scientific Revolutions*. Chicago: Chicago Press.

Lisle, J. (1991). Workplace transformations. In P. Draper (ed.), *Health Through Public Policy*. London: Green Print.

Lisle, J. R. & Newsome A (1989). Health promotion and counselling. *Occupational Health Practice*, 3rd edn. London: Butterworth and Company.

Lisle, J. & Watkins, S. (1991). Healthier and safer workplaces. In P. Draper (ed.), *Health Through Public Policy*. London: Green Print.

National Health Service Executive (1994). *Health Promoting Hospitals*. London: Department of Health.

Office of Population Censuses and Surveys (1992). *Labour Force Survey 1990 and 1991*. Series LFS no. 9. London: HMSO.

Schilling, R. S. F. (1989). Health protection and promotion at work. *British Journal of Industrial Medicine*, 46(10), 683–688.

World Health Organisation (1990). *Occupational Health Services – An Overview*. Regional Publications European Series 26. Copenhagen: WHO.

World Health Organisation (1993). *Health for All Targets. The Health Policy for Europe*. Updated edition, September 1991. Copenhagen: WHO.

Wynne, R. (1990). *Innovative Workplace Actions for Health: An Overview of the Situation in Seven European Countries*. Dublin: Work Research Centre.

Wynne, R. & Clarkin, N. (1992). *European Foundation for the Improvement of Living and Working Conditions. Under Construction – Building for Health in the EC Workplace*. Luxembourg: Office for Official Publications of the European Communities.

Author index

Subject index